Copyright Information

Disclaimer

Table of Contents

I. Too Good to Be True?

They say that the only place where "fat melts right off your body" is in the ads... especially the ones for those diet products you see on late night TV. So, I guess this is where I should tone down my original claims (i.e. the ones made on my website that prompted you to buy this book) and give it to you straight...

Except... that's not going to happen. You see, unlike any other diet product – be it a book, pill, shake, or any of those infomercial contraptions you may have purchased in the past... this one stands true to its word.

There's no need to tone down anything. That's because **if you follow the simple advice written in these pages you *will* lose weight faster (and easier) than you ever dreamed possible.** That's no exaggeration either. Best of all, you'll keep it off for the rest of your life. And that's a promise.

Now, I can understand your skepticism. After all, weight loss is "supposed" to be hard, right? You need strength, determination, and monumental willpower to get and stay skinny. More specifically, you need to watch your calories, control your portions, keep track of carbs, and make sure you eat every few hours so your metabolism doesn't crash.

And let's not forget: you need to starve yourself, exercise for hours on end, give up your favorite foods... and eat nothing but a bland diet for the rest of your life. And then maybe (*if your metabolism isn't already "shot"*)... maybe... you have a chance at slimming down.

Does that sound about right?

Well, I'm here to tell you that nothing could be further from the truth. Of course, you'd never know it by taking a quick look around you. Everywhere you turn, you see people who are either overweight or even clinically obese.

And it's a shame. Because as far as I'm concerned, it's not their fault. You see, *most* of the people who have given us dietary advice throughout the years are dead wrong. Not all, but most.

It's a strong statement, I know. But it's either that or there's some big conspiracy going on. I'd like to believe it's the former. But unfortunately, that can't be the case... at least not entirely.

Listen, **the diet industry needs you to stay fat**. They need you to be confused. Why? So they can keep selling you more products. More books and magazines, more pills, more powders, more meals, more contraptions, etc., etc., etc...

If you can get and stay slim by eating nothing but the right foods, entire industries would instantly dry up. The diet industry? POOF... gone in an instant. Billions of dollars in profits would vanish into thin air.

And how about Big Pharma? What if everyone were thin? We'd have just a tiny fraction of the diseases we have today. Heartburn, heart disease, cancer, Alzheimer's (to name a few) are all linked to obesity in one way or another. And the pharmaceutical companies make *billions* peddling their pills that only mask the symptoms yet do nothing to solve the underlying problem.

Now, I realize I'm going off on a tangent. After all, this is supposed to be a diet book. But in fact, it's a little more than that. And when you're done reading it, I want you to be able to look at the world of health and nutrition in a different light.

That's because...

I don't just want you to be thin. I want you to have the best health humanly possible. More importantly, I want you to be in total control of that health. That only comes with education.

The information that follows is very powerful. Use it to your greatest advantage. By doing so, not only will you look and feel better than you've had in years (perhaps ever) – you'll also be better educated about nutrition than 99% of the population. And again, that education is power which puts total control of your health *in your hands* – not your doctor's or anyone else's.

Now, before we get started let me apologize in advance. Why?

Because I'm not a professional writer. So, if you're reading this for its literary style I'm afraid you'll be disappointed. I write like I talk and my only concern is that my message makes an impact on your life – nothing more.

Again, for this, I am sorry...

And one final thing before we get started: **you MUST read this book from cover to cover. Please do not SKIP to any single page**. Here's why: the nuts and bolts of this program are in Chapter VI. However, the pages leading up to that are arguably the most important of the book. They explain why you're doing what you're doing based on hard science.

Why do you need to know that?

Because... if you don't understand the concepts behind this diet you'll never see it through... and ultimately, fail. I don't want you to make that mistake and rob yourself of the chance to have the body (and health) you've always wanted.

So again, please read this from cover to cover. Now, let's begin...

II. Why We Got Into This Mess in the First Place

Weight gain was always a growing problem throughout history. But by the late 70's it began reaching epidemic proportions. Today, two-thirds of Americans are overweight while a good portion of them are clinically obese.

And if you were to ask ten different people why that is, you'd likely get different responses (fast food, stress, lack of sleep, a slow metabolism, no time to work out, etc.). However, the general consensus would revolve around diet and exercise. More specifically, that we eat too much and don't move enough... or as the Bible refers to it: gluttony and sloth.

And while that's true to some degree, it doesn't explain why the rate of obesity began to skyrocket *at one specific point in time*: the late 70's. Why not before? I mean, did we just wake up one day and collectively decide to become gluttonous sloths?

It doesn't seem rational, does it? After all, I don't know *anyone* who chooses to be fat? Do you? So in light of this, perhaps something else is to blame besides our laziness" and "lack of willpower".

Well, as it turns out... there is.

In fact, there's a very simple explanation as to why this all happened. It started in 1957 with a scientist by the name of Ancel Keys. Now, Keys was on a crusade against saturated fat. He was convinced that it was the root cause of all our health problems, and specifically, heart disease.

So, he set out to do what any good scientist does when they have a theory: he conducted a study to see if he could prove it. And he did. After analyzing the eating habits of people from seven different countries, Keys concluded that the more saturated fat one ate, the higher their blood levels of cholesterol, and the higher their incidence of heart disease.

His findings were irrefutable. In fact, when the data from the seven countries was plotted on a graph, the points formed a straight line... as straight as straight could get.

And so, the "lipid hypothesis" was born. Keys got himself on the cover of Time Magazine and the government stepped in to advise us, Americans, about how we should eat to prevent disease.

A committee was formed led by Senator George McGovern. Its goal was to set nutritional guidelines for the public in an effort to fight what were becoming far too common conditions: high blood pressure, diabetes, strokes, heart attacks, etc... Of course, based on Keys' findings, their recommendation was to dramatically lower the amount of fat and cholesterol in our diet.

Now, it's worth noting that at the time, several scientists spoke out against these guidelines, citing the need to conduct further research. The committee did, in fact, have very little to go on... despite their reception of Keys' findings with open arms.

Unfortunately their pleas fell on deaf ears. And in January of 1977 *"Dietary Goals for the United States"* (also known as the McGovern report) was released to the American public. The USDA also stepped in to give us our recommended food pyramid.

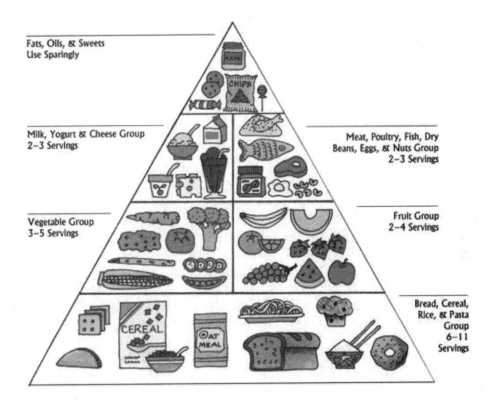

The rest, of course, is history. Fat became our sworn enemy. And if we were to stay healthy, we needed to replace the calories that previously came from fats, with several servings of carbohydrates: bread, cereal, pasta, etc...

Now, this should have solved our health problems... but as you can see on the following graph, it obviously didn't. As stated previously, we started gaining weight like there was no tomorrow. Just look at what happened right around 1980!

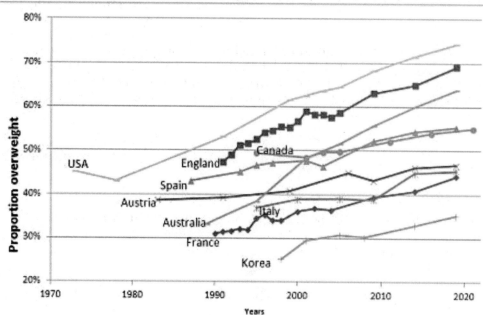

Past and projected future overweight rates in selected OECD countries

And do you want to know why?

Because Keys' study was bogus. It's not Time Magazine he should have been in… but jail! You see, it was later discovered that he had studied not seven but twenty-two countries. And when THAT data was plotted on a graph, the points were all over the place. In other words, **there was no correlation between the saturated fat in one's diet and their incidence of heart disease**.

But Keys was so hell-bent on proving his theory, he disregarded all the data that didn't support his hypothesis. And millions upon millions of people have paid – *and continue to pay* – the ultimate price for that (you'll understand why shortly).

But in all fairness, Keys and the McGovern committee aren't the only ones to blame for our obesity epidemic. Scores of scientists with tunnel vision just as bad as theirs have bombarded us with plenty of false information since then.

Perhaps the most damaging of our current times is the following…

III. A Calorie is a Calorie is a Calorie... or is It?

Everyone knows that in order to lose weight you must burn more calories than you consume. So if you eat, let's say... 500 fewer calories per day than you need to maintain your current weight, you *should* lose about a pound of fat per week (note: a pound of fat is made up of 3,500 calories, so 500 x 7 days = 3,500).

Furthermore, as far as weight loss is concerned, it doesn't' matter *where* those calories come from. As long as "calories in" is less than "calories out", you'll lose weight.

Now, the above has been the topic of intense debate for some time. So, in order to set the record straight, Kansas State University nutrition professor, Mark Haub, decided to go on a diet. But not just any diet... a diet consisting of nothing more than Twinkies and donuts.

What happened?

Surprisingly, he lost 27 pounds in 2 months. He also dropped his LDL ("bad") cholesterol by 20%, upped his HDL ("good") cholesterol by 20%, and reduced his triglycerides by 39%.

Pretty impressive... considering the fact that he was eating nothing but junk food, don't you think?

It also proves that a calorie *is* just a calorie. In other words, it doesn't matter where your food comes from (i.e. carbohydrates, proteins, fats). As long as you consume fewer calories than your body needs to maintain "energy balance"... you'll lose weight.

In Professor Haub's case, he needed ~ 2,600 calories/day to maintain his weight. He only ate 1,800 creating a deficit of 800. And voila... easy weight loss.

Now mind you, he made it very clear that *nobody* should follow his diet (it's officially called *The Twinkie Diet*). I don't understand why. After all, didn't his markers of health improve dramatically?

It's this kind of disconnect that really irks me. You have a professor (of nutrition, no less) going on national TV and broadcasting to millions of people how he was able to lose weight by eating calories from junk food. And then... he tells you to eat healthy calories.

So, which one is it? Do we need quality calories to lose weight and improve health or not?

Regardless of how he might answer this question, you have to take the following into consideration: **his experiment is extremely misleading**. Why? Because **it won't work for everybody. In fact, it probably won't work for *a lot* people** (e.g. put a diabetic on this plan and you'll quickly send them to the grave).

The only reason it worked for him is because he still had a "functional metabolism" (we'll discuss this in detail shortly). It may not have been perfect. After all, he was overweight at the beginning of the experiment. But it was good enough to enable weight loss despite a diet of junk food.

Now, if he *didn't* have a functional (*or at least a partially functional*) metabolism, he could have cut his calories to a mere 1,200 day and he would have lost very little weight, if any, on a diet of fat and sugar.

How can I be so sure?

Because, I also followed a low-calorie diet that was relatively high in sugar. For 12 weeks I ate a low-fat diet consisting mainly of "healthy" carbs (*keep in mind that all carbs are essentially broken down into simple sugar for digestion*), very little meat, and a lot of fruit. I also exercised six times a week.

I needed around 2,800 calories/day to maintain my weight. I ate an average of 2,000. I know this because I kept track of what I was eating in a food journal. It was awful. Nevertheless, I should have been losing about 1.5 pounds/week based on the calories in-calories out equation (or approximately 18 total by the end of the 12 weeks that I was on my diet).

Total weight lost? **ZERO.** The scale literally did not budge.

And what's worse is that I was hungry the entire time (the nighttime cravings were unbearable). Not to mention, I deprived myself of most of the foods I loved and it was all for nothing.

So what changed? And how was I able to drop 36 pounds in the following 2 months... almost effortlessly? Simple. I turned my dysfunctional metabolism into a functional one (*a very functional one at that*).

How?

I cut down on starch and simple sugars (you'll learn why, exactly, in the next chapter). Not entirely, mind you... but enough to make a *drastic* difference to my metabolism. By day 3 on my "new diet" I felt an unbelievable amount of energy. And by day 10 I started losing weight very, very fast.

The best part?

I ate like a pig (no exaggeration). I didn't count calories or keep track of anything. I exercised *zero* portion control. I was never hungry and I never felt deprived. And the weight still kept coming off – just by keeping my sugar intake to a minimum.

So how is that possible?

How can someone fail to lose weight (or lose very little) on a low-calorie diet but literally "melt away" the pounds on a high calorie diet?

Because **a calorie IS NOT just a calorie. It matters *where* your food comes from – a lot. And that goes double if your metabolism isn't working.**

That is the reason why most people can't lose meaningful amounts of weight. We're told over and over again to read food labels... to make sure we're not eating too many calories – particularly too many calories from fat.

But instead of focusing on total calories and fat – you should be focusing on sugar. The less you consume, the better.

Why?

In one word: **insulin**. As you may already know, insulin is a hormone secreted by the pancreas in response to rising levels of blood glucose (i.e. sugar). It's absolutely *crucial* for survival because too much blood sugar is toxic. So, every time you eat a meal that contains sugar, insulin is responsible for moving that sugar from your bloodstream into your tissues (e.g. muscle, liver, etc.).

The higher the sugar content of your meal, the more insulin you'll secrete. And when you take the dietary recommendations set forth by the USDA and combine them with the "lesson" of Mark Haub's experiment, you create the perfect storm.

Here's why...

When insulin levels are elevated, you cannot burn fat. That's because insulin inhibits an enzyme present on your fat cells known as hormone sensitive lipase (HSL). In the absence of insulin, this enzyme burns fat to provide your cells with energy... **but not when insulin levels are high**.

Now, do you see why it's important to restrict sugar?

And as mentioned above, all carbohydrates are essentially sugar. It doesn't matter if you eat white bread or whole grains. Eventually, they all get broken down into sugar. The only reason whole grains are preferred is because they contain a lot of fiber. As a result, they don't cause as much of an insulin spike as a piece of candy would.

So, am I telling you to eliminate all carbohydrates from your diet? Of course not. That's neither desirable – nor necessary. However, you *will* need to restrict them somewhat if you're having trouble losing weight, have elevated cholesterol levels, blood pressure, blood sugar, etc...

But even though you'll need to exercise a tiny bit of restraint, I'll show you how you can keep eating all your favorite foods and still have an excellent metabolism. Furthermore, by the time we go over all of the concepts in this program, everything will make perfect sense. You won't have to think about any of this – it will become second nature. That's the beauty of this: it's effortless while at the same time extremely effective.

Now, before we move on to the next chapter, I'd like to take a moment to *really* drive that last point home because it's **the secret to permanent weight loss. It will also explain why you may have failed to achieve this in the past by following plans such as Weight Watchers** (i.e. ones that allow you to eat anything you want provided you don't exceed your daily or weekly points).

Please take a look at the image on the next page...

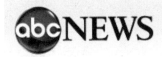

Low-Cal Peanut Butter Is a Dream for Dieters

By Lauren Torrisi | ABC News Blogs – 21 hrs ago

Email   Recommend 10   Tweet 2   Share   Print

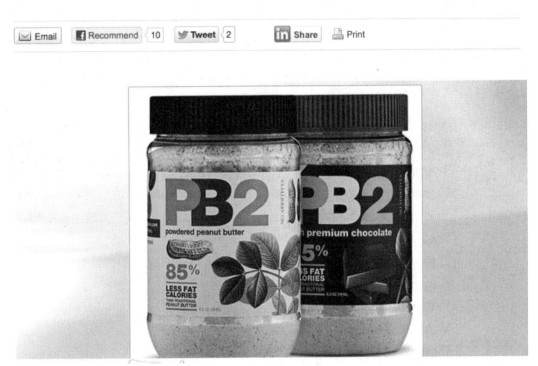

It's a screenshot of an article showcasing a new peanut butter some company recently concocted. By removing the fat they've reduced the calories per serving from the normal 190 to a mere 45! Now on the surface, this may seem like a dieter's dream (as the article's title suggests). But rest assured, this is the stuff that nightmares are truly made of.

The reason why can be found in the following two screenshots: the first one is the nutrition facts of PB2, the low-calorie, low-fat peanut butter. The second one is the nutrition facts of my favorite all-natural peanut butter, Teddy.

Nutrition facts:

PB2: Powdered Peanut Butter

Ingredients: Roasted peanuts, sugar and salt.

Serving size: 2 Tablespoons (12 grams)

Servings per container: 15

Calories: 45

Calories from fat: 13

Value and % Daily Value*

Total fat 1.5 g 3%

Saturated fat 0 g 0%

Trans fat < 0.01 g

Cholesterol < 0.01 mg 0%

Sodium 94 mg 4%

Total carbohydrate 5 g 2%

Dietary fiber 2 g 8%

Sugars 1 g

Protein 5 g

Vitamin A < 1%

Vitamin C 0%

Calcium <1%

Iron 0%

*Percent Daily Values are based on a 2000 calorie diet.

Details	All Natural Super Chunky	All Natural Super Chunky UNSALTED	All Natural Smooth	All Natural Smooth UNSALTED
INGREDIENTS	Roasted Peanuts, Salt	Roasted Peanuts	Roasted Peanuts, Salt	Roasted Peanuts
Calories	190	190	190	190
Fat Calories	140	140	140	140
Total Fat	16g	16g	16g	16g
Sat. Fat	2g	2g	2g	2g
Trans Fat	0g	0g	0g	0g
Polyunsat. Fat	5g	5g	5g	5g
Monounsat. Fat	8g	8g	8g	8g
Cholesterol	0mg	0mg	0mg	0mg
Sodium	100mg	0mg	125mg	0mg
Total Carb	7g	7g	7g	7g
Fiber	3g	3g	3g	3g
Sugars	1g	1g	1g	1g
Protein	8g	8g	8g	8g
Percent Daily Values are based on a 2,000 calorie diet.	Calcium 2% Iron 4% Vitamin E 10% Folate 10% Niacin 20%	Calcium 2% Iron 4% Vitamin E 10% Folate 10% Niacin 20%	Calcium 2% Iron 4% Vitamin E 10% Folate 10% Niacin 20%	Calcium 2% Iron 4% Vitamin E 10% Folate 10% Niacin 20%

Alright, let's take a closer look at these labels:

- PB2 calories per serving: 45; Teddy calories per serving: 190.
- PB2 carbs and sugar: 5 and 1 (respectively); Teddy carbs and sugar: 7 and 1 (respectively).

So, at first glance, it almost seems obvious that the PB2 would be a better choice if you were dieting. After all, fewer calories consumed = faster fat loss, right? And on paper that's entirely true. Unfortunately, that's not how things play out in real life (and the reason why the majority of dieters fail to lose weight and/or keep it off long-term).

Let me explain...

Study after study has shown that people who opt for these low-fat, low-calorie foods always overeat. And there are a couple of reasons for this:

1. They feel less guilt about doing so because, after all, "it's low in calories".

2. More importantly, they don't get the same satisfaction or feeling of fullness the way they would if they ate the non-diet, full-fat counterpart.

Now let's examine the second point in a little more detail because it forms the basis of this argument (and again, the key to permanent weight loss)...

In our peanut butter example, if you were to eat 2 tablespoons of the Teddy, you'd get very full – very fast (I know this to be true because I'd eat it every night to fight my cravings while I was on one of my low-fat, calorie-counting diets). 2 tablespoons were more than enough for a (then) 200+ pound man.

But 2 tablespoons of the PB2 would not be nearly enough. Why?

Simple: because it has very little fat. And on the surface, this seems like a good thing. However, fat plays a very important role in nature: it makes us feel full. Without it, you can't achieve that same level of satiety and you crave more.

So, instead of settling for 2 tablespoons (i.e. 1 serving), you'd need 5 or 6 (i.e. 3 servings) to get the same level of fullness. And even then, you *still* wouldn't achieve the same effect (explained below).

But what's the big deal, you might be asking yourself? Even if you *did* eat 6 tablespoons of the PB2 you'd still have eaten only 135 calories vs. the 190 from the Teddy. And while that's true, here's where that "calorie is a calorie" debate comes into the equation.

6 tablespoons of PB2 would net you 135 calories, 15 grams of carbohydrates, 3 grams of sugar, and 4.5 grams of fat (also 282 mg. of sodium; hello hypertension). On the other hand, 2 tablespoons of Teddy would net you 190 calories, 7 grams of carbohydrates, 1 gram of sugar, and 16 grams of fat.

Now because the former is stripped of almost all fat it won't keep you full for very long. Therefore, you're more likely to seek out something else to eat in a short while to curb your cravings. So in the end, you end up eating more calories – just not in one sitting.

The only way to prevent this from happening is to exercise willpower. When those new cravings arise you have to *consciously* fight them so you don't go over your daily calories, points, or any other restrictive system you happen to be on.

On the contrary, the Teddy has plenty of fat (naturally) and will keep you satisfied much longer. Sure, you may be eating more calories in one sitting, but you're eating fewer calories overall.

In the first scenario you're relying on willpower to achieve weight loss while in the second you're relying on instinct – your natural survival instinct to keep you fed and satisfied. Now, if you had to bet on the above two (i.e. willpower vs. instinct)... which do you think would win in the long run?

Take a moment to think about that because, again, it's the key to rapid and _permanent_ weight loss.

Let's move on...

When foods are stripped of their natural fat to make them less caloric, they end up tasting really bad. In order to compensate for this, manufacturers add salt and sugar. As you already know, salt is linked to high blood pressure. It's bad stuff in big quantities. And sugar is no saint either. As mentioned previously, having more than a teaspoon in your bloodstream will make you very sick – it can even kill you.

Luckily insulin prevents this from happening by clearing it from your bloodstream. But aside from that, it also pushes fat into your fat cells. And, if you remember from above, **it prevents fat from being released into your bloodstream to be used for energy.**

And the latter point is another reason why dieters are always hungry. They have plenty of energy stored as body fat, but high levels of insulin won't let them use it. As a result, they need to eat every few hours or they'll feel tired and cranky. And this just repeats the above process: more sugar results in higher levels of insulin, more fat going into fat cells, and the inability to use that fat for energy.

So again, even though one food provides you with fewer calories, you're forced to eat it more often because your body craves nutrients. The end result? Inevitable weight gain.

Now, if you've ever been on a program such as Weight Watchers, no doubt you've experienced this. That's because, in order to please you, they allow you to eat whatever you want (provided it's portion controlled and doesn't exceed your points). And sure, you can lose weight this way. Thousands of people do. But how many of them keep it off? Ever been to a meeting before? How many of the attendees are starting the program for the second, third, or fourth time?

And again, the reason is simple: if you eat the right foods, you won't have to exercise willpower, count points, calories, or exercise portion control. Your body is perfectly capable of letting you know when and how much to eat (i.e.

natural instinct). This way losing weight and keeping it off becomes second nature.

On the other hand, if you eat the wrong foods, you're on your own. You have to count, calculate, and track – not to mention exercise willpower to fight the inevitable cravings (i.e. your body's way of telling you it's missing nutrients). And how long can you expect to fight and hunger... and win?

If you can truly grasp this concept you'll go on to lose all of your extra weight both quickly and easily... the same way I did and thousands of followers of this program.

Alright, with that out of the way, let's move on to what is, perhaps, the most important chapter in this entire book. So, pay very close attention to what I'm about to reveal to you...

IV. The Paradigm Shift

Shortly after my final dieting attempt (which as you know, failed miserably) I made a discovery that changed my life forever. *This* is what allowed me to lose all of my extra weight – practically effortlessly – and become healthier than I've ever been. And since then, I've never looked back.

Here's what happened...

I was browsing online looking for something – *anything* – that would help me get back on the wagon. That's when I came across a book called "Why We Get Fat: And What to Do About It" by science writer Gary Taubes. I read the first few pages via Amazon's preview feature and I was hooked. Not wanting to wait for it to arrive by mail, I rushed to Barnes & Noble to buy it.

> **SIDENOTE:** By the way, you should **get yourself a copy of this book**. In fact, get several and give them to your friends and family as gifts.... and even one for your doctor.

Getting back to the story... I started reading the book immediately. And about a third of the way in, **I came to a sentence that stopped me dead in my tracks**. This was one of the biggest "AHA" moments I had ever had... and my weight (and health) has never been an issue since then.

So what was it?

"We don't get fat because we overeat – We overeat because we're getting fat."

As you can see, it's a complete paradigm shift and turns a near-universal view on its head. So read it again, several times, and let it sink in.

Now, in the book he goes on to explain why that is the case. He provides plenty of evidence, both anecdotal and hard science. But two of the arguments that really stuck with me are the following...

1. When you're young and going through your growth spurt, you're obviously gaining weight. You're also eating more. However, you're not growing taller because you're taking in more calories. You're taking in more calories because you're growing taller.

    More specifically, your body is releasing a range of hormones (e.g. Growth Hormone, Testosterone, T3/T4, etc.). And it's because of those hormones that you eat more than you previously did. The causation is reversed. Sure, the food is required for growth, but the only reason you're inclined to eat more is because your hormones are commanding you to.

The same goes for weight gain beyond your growth spurt. Your hormones are commanding you to eat more – not your lack of willpower.

2. He talked about experiments done on obesogenic mice. These are mice that have been genetically altered to gain weight easily. They are commonly used to study the effects of different diets and other behaviors on weight loss/gain.

   And in one particular experiment, the mice were starved to death. Now, one would assume that since they weren't being fed, they would eat their own fat stores to stay alive. But that wasn't the case. In fact, when the autopsies were conducted, the mice had preserved most of their fat stores... *at the expense of eating their muscles, and eventually their heart for fuel.*

   In other words, they cannibalized their vital organs so they wouldn't need to burn off fat. They didn't choose to do this. But obviously, their hormonal state (due to their genetic alteration) wouldn't allow them to use fat for fuel.

And as you'll soon discover, this is largely what happens to people without a functional metabolism... and... the reason why it's so difficult to lose meaningful amounts of weight by simply eating less and exercising more.

If you're a bit confused, don't worry. This will all make perfect sense when these concepts are tied together in the following chapter.

V. How to "Reset" Your Metabolism for Effortless Weight Loss

Alright, in the previous chapters we discussed the function of insulin and how it essentially regulates weight gain. To recap: it's responsible for clearing sugar from your bloodstream and also shuttles fat into fat cells.

We also noted that the higher the sugar content of a meal, the more insulin gets secreted from your pancreas. And finally, the higher your levels of insulin, the less fat you're able to burn for energy (if you recall, insulin prevents the release of fatty acids from your fat cells by inhibiting the enzyme "hormone sensitive lipase" or HSL).

Now, when you're young, you need very little insulin to clear sugar from your bloodstream. That's because your cells (e.g. muscle, liver) are still "sensitive" to its effects.

In contrast, as you get older you become insulin resistant. The result? You need a lot *more* insulin to clear sugar from your bloodstream. And as noted above, more insulin equals more fat storage.

That's the reason why some people can eat whatever they want and never gain an ounce. Their cells are very responsive to insulin even as they get older. On the other end of the spectrum, when someone's cells become extremely resistant to insulin, they can't clear sugar from their bloodstream and eventually become diabetic.

Stated differently, the former has a functional (or fast) metabolism while the latter has a dysfunctional (or slow) metabolism. And sure, genetics play a key role in this. However, if you're not blessed with "great genes" (few people are) you can easily "reset" your metabolism so that it becomes functional once again.

How?

Simple: **keep your insulin levels as low as possible!**

And not only because high levels of insulin make you fat. They're also responsible for causing heart disease, high blood pressure, cancer, Alzheimer's, and most other "chronic diseases of aging".

> **SIDENOTE:** You can find mountains of information and published studies on the above by Googling "insulin heart disease" or "insulin Alzheimer's", etc...

Now, how do you keep your insulin levels as low as possible? Again, you limit the amount of carbohydrates in your diet (*this, plus a meal-timing method that will literally melt fat right off your body; discussed later*).

If you recall from chapter III, all carbohydrates are eventually broken down into simple sugars for digestion. However, not all carbohydrates evoke the same insulin response (and hence, not all are bad for you).

As a rule of thumb, the higher the fiber content of a carbohydrate – the lower the insulin response (fiber prevents rapid rises in blood sugar). Now, here are some examples of the best to worst carbohydrates in decreasing order:

1. **Vegetables**. These have a very high fiber content and result in a minimal insulin response. They're also packed with vitamins, minerals, and antioxidants. These should be the staple of your everyday diet.

2. **Fruit**. Like vegetables, fruit is also packed with vitamins, minerals, and antioxidants. But in contrast to the former, fruit contains a lot of sugar. As such, this food gets a "mixed blessing". Moderation is key.

3. **Whole grains** (e.g. oatmeal). Not anywhere near as good for you as the USDA would have you believe. Still, they're better than refined carbs due to their high fiber content. Unfortunately, they're a major source of calories in our diet contributing to our epidemic of obesity and diabetes.

4. **Refined carbs** (e.g. white bread, white rice). Very insulinogenic. Avoid as much as possible due to their low fiber content.

5. **Fruit juices.** Contrary to popular belief, juice is *not* good for you. Why? It's a matter of volume. When you drink a glass of orange juice, you're ingesting several oranges at once (and a boatload of sugar). Furthermore, it lacks the fiber you would normally get if you were eating the fruit whole so your blood sugar rises very fast after drinking it.

6. **Candy, cookies, cakes, and other sweets.** These should be avoided like the plague except on special occasions (explained later). They contain too much sugar and "artery-clogging" trans-fats.

7. **Soda.** If you're a soda drinker, one of the fastest ways to lose weight and start getting healthier is to replace soda with water. Soda is arguably one of the major contributors to our obesity and diabetes epidemic worldwide.

OK, now that you have a general idea of what causes weight gain, I'd like to revisit the calories-in/calories-out discussion so that you can truly understand why limiting sugar in your diet will lead to effortless weight loss despite eating "as much as you want".

Let's start by examining the following equations:

$$\Delta_{ENERGY} = E_{IN} - E_{OUT}$$

This is the first law of thermodynamics. It states that energy in a closed system is constant. It can neither be created nor destroyed – just transferred. And, applied to weight maintenance it becomes the following:

$$\Delta_{WEIGHT} = CALORIES_{IN} - CALORIES_{OUT}$$

In essence, weight loss/gain/maintenance is a direct result of how many calories you consume via food minus how many you burn via exercise (and of course, normal cellular activity).

But wait a minute...

Didn't we say that this is not the case when we discussed Professor Haub? And that if you don't have a functional metabolism... you can't eat the wrong foods (*even in small amounts*) and expect to lose weight?

Now here's where it gets interesting. **The first law of thermodynamics is immutable. And weight loss *is* a result of calories in minus calories out. However, that equation doesn't take one very important factor into account: _how your body decides to use those calories_.**

Let me explain by painting you a picture...

Let's say that you sit down to eat a big, 1,000 calorie, high carbohydrate meal... a huge overflowing plate of mouth-watering pasta topped with a mountain of marinara sauce and 2 gigantic, juicy, meatballs.

And after scarfing it all down, you start feeling "heavy". So you make your way to the couch and turn on the TV. About 15 minutes later you've dosed off only to wake up hungry in a couple of hours. You give in to your cravings and decide to eat some cookies.

Now, what has happened here?

It's simple. The high carb content of the pasta caused your blood sugar to spike. As a result, your pancreas started pumping insulin like crazy to get the sugar out of your bloodstream (remember, it's toxic at high levels). Some of it went into your muscles and liver to be stored as glycogen. But their storage capacity is very limited.

What happened to the rest? **It went right into your fat cells and was converted to fat**. And unlike your muscles or your liver, your fat tissue has *unlimited* storage capacity.

Now here's where things really start to break down...

Because your insulin spiked as a result of the high carb load, it overcorrected and decreased your blood sugar levels too much. The result? You started feeling hungry again even though you ate a huge meal a couple of hours ago. **The energy is still there but you can't use it**. It's locked inside your fat cells because your high insulin levels won't let it out.

Now let's look at a different scenario...

Instead of a high carb meal, you decide to eat a big piece of salmon with a heaping portion of crunchy asparagus. Like the other meal, this too was about 1,000 calories. But this time, that heavy feeling of digestion is non-existent. You get up from the table and go do some yard work. Furthermore, you don't even think about food for several hours because you feel so full.

Let's examine the difference in a little more detail...

Because you didn't eat large amount of carbs, your insulin didn't spike. As a result, your body was free to feed off the fat and protein content of the fish. And... once you burned that off (remember, instead of taking a nap you felt energetic and went out to work on your lawn) your body was able to use your stored fat as energy.

Same amount of calories consumed – much different result...

In the first scenario you'd end up gaining weight. Remember, you were hungry when you woke up from your nap and had to eat *again*. And I don't know about you, but after large pasta meals I crave sweets due to the resulting low blood sugar from the insulin spike. But in the second scenario you felt full, satisfied, and very energetic. Furthermore, you weren't hungry for hours.

This is why attempting portion control or trying to count calories doesn't work. It's even worse when you add exercise into the mix. Look, your body is much smarter than you think. It's the most amazing creation in existence. It has several redundant systems to maintain homeostasis. And… **it doesn't want to be fat.**

If you feed it what it needs, you never have to worry about overeating. If you happen to eat "more than you should" during one meal, you'll feel a burst of energy that will cause you to move and burn these calories off.

You literally will not be able to just sit on the couch and watch TV (if you recall from a previous chapter, this is the exact reason why I started feeling tremendous amounts of energy on or around the 3rd day of modifying my diet).

Now let's wrap this up…

Energy in (or eating) and Energy out (or exercise) are interlinked. If you don't eat enough… or eat the wrong foods… your body will start starving and decrease your movements. You'll feel tired and want to rest.

On the contrary, if you overeat your body will feel the need to burn off that extra energy and cause you to move more. Not to mention that it's not possible to overeat when you're eating the right foods (that is, unless you force yourself).

Like everything else, your body knows when it wants to stop – you don't have to exercise restraint. In other words, things go back to the way nature intended them to be: **hunger and eating should be instinctual processes – not intellectual!**

Really simple, isn't it?

Now let's get down to the nuts and bolts of this program…

VI. The Nuts and Bolts of the Cruise Control Diet

A. Overview

If you've been around the diet game for some time then this is probably starting to look like your typical low-carb plan like Atkins or South Beach. However, I assure you that it's not.

Of course, you *will* find many similarities with the above mentioned. After all, I didn't invent this stuff and would never dream of taking full credit for it. However, a lot of credit *does* go to Dr. Atkins for his work in the field of metabolism and the carbohydrate's effect on it.

He really tried to open our eyes but was sadly shunned for it by the medical establishment. Luckily, that's slowly changing. And in the future, you're going to see a much wider acceptance of these concepts.

With that said, here's why The Cruise Control Diet is unique in its own right: it becomes an afterthought. It doesn't rely on counting carbs or calories or any type of portion control. In fact, you don't have to calculate or keep track of anything. As mentioned in the previous chapter, the process becomes instinctual – not intellectual.

And that's very important because very few people can give that much emphasis to the mathematics of nutrition for any appreciable amount of time... and hence, why they can't stay on the diets that led them to lose weight long-term.

It's safe to assume that you aren't one of those outliers – otherwise you probably wouldn't be reading this right now. You'd already have the body you currently want.

With this in mind, you'll find my eating plan much more suited to your needs. It takes everything we've just discussed into account and puts it into practice so that you don't have to think about how and when to eat... ever. It also prevents you from binging by virtually eliminating your cravings.

However, that's not to say that you won't binge. In fact, I encourage it from time to time. That's right, you can still eat the chocolate, the cakes, the chips, and all that other stuff I just told you that you shouldn't. Furthermore, when you get rolling on this diet – not only will it NOT hurt your progress... it will actually help it (more on that later).

So, now that you know what you won't be doing... what is it that you *will* be doing?

Simple... you're going to listen to your body (what a concept, right?) **You're going to eat when you're hungry and you won't when you're not. In short, the primary tool you'll use to lose all of your extra weight (*and keep it off for good*) is hunger...**

Now, you may be thinking to yourself that your appetite led you to pack on the pounds in the first place. So, how could listening to your hunger signals possibly help? Well, the reason you gained weight to begin with was because of your dysfunctional metabolism.

Remember, your body does not want to be fat. And before we get into the mechanics of why this is the case... consider the following...

In our roughly 2.5 millions years of evolution, we've only been eating starches and grains for the last 10,000 years or so. This is when all of our problems began.

You see, prior to this, we didn't know much (if anything) about calories and macronutrients. We just ate when we were hungry (and when food was available). Yet, we never *really* gained weight – at least not for any appreciable amount of time.

The same holds true for animals. If you exclude our domestic pets like cats and dogs that eat unnatural carb loaded processed foods... wild animals never get fat. And do you know why? Because they have a functional metabolism – a direct result of them eating the diet they evolved to eat for millions of years.

Now, here's what happens when you eat the way nature intended you to eat and you reset your metabolism...

1. You'll switch from being a sugar burner to a fat burner. Because your insulin levels will drop, HSL – the enzyme present on your fat cells – will not be blocked. This will allow it to release free fatty acids into your bloodstream. As a result, not only will you lose weight, you'll also experience a surge in energy. And more movement = greater calorie burn = faster weight loss.

2. You'll stop getting hungry every 2-3 hours and the cravings will virtually vanish. That means you won't have to eat 5-6 small meals per day – or 3 meals and 2 snacks... or any of that other nonsense nutritionists have been touting for years.

And don't worry, your metabolism won't "crash" like you've been warned. You'll also never get the shakes or feel jittery because you've gone for too long without food.

In fact, you'll never again feel hunger the way you do now (that is, the way you do now on the typical high-carb meal). Instead, hunger will set in very slowly and your energy levels won't suddenly drop.

At this point, I feel compelled to interject with the following tidbit concerning the myth that your metabolism will slow down if you don't eat every few hours. If this was truly the case, I would have never written this and you wouldn't be reading it right now.

Why?

Because the lions would have wiped us out many, many years ago. Can you imagine if our physiology was that inefficient so as to not allow us to function without food in our stomach for more than a few hours? What about the times when prehistoric man went out on hunts and returned empty handed.

How did he survive?

Again, by asking these questions you get to see how little thought is given to the recommendations made by the "experts". Now, in all fairness, as a sugar burner, you really can't go without food for too long without getting weak. But that's not how nature intended you to be. Our body's primary preference is to burn fat – not sugar.

Nevertheless, now's a good time to dispel yet another myth concerning multiple meals a day. We've been told that the more frequently you eat, the more calories you burn to digest that meal. This is known as the thermic effect of food or TEF.

Basically, 10% of the calories in any given meal are burned off during the digestion process. So the "logic" is – eat more often to burn more calories.

But consider this: if you ate a total of 3,000 calories per day divided over 6 meals, you'd be consuming 500 calories per meal and burning 50 of those for digestion (10% of 500 = 50). So, over the course of your 6 meals you'd burn a total of 300 calories (50 x 6 = 300).

Now, what if instead of 6 meals of 500, you ate 3 meals of 1000? Well, you'd use 10% of your 1,000-calorie meal for digestion, or 100 calories. And 100 x 3 = 300. As you can see the thermic effect of food is the same regardless of how many meals you eat.

Here's the bottom line: eat as many times as you feel like. If you want to eat 6 times a day, so be it. If you're real busy and don't have the time, fine – eat 2 or 3 times. That's the beauty of this program. It completely fits into your lifestyle.

3. And finally, when you eat the way nature intended you to, you'll stop overeating. In other words, you'll find the perfect caloric balance without counting, calculating, or weighing food.

   Your body knows how much to eat better than any derived and rigid formula that a diet guru comes up with. For example, there's a diet (I won't mention names) that makes you eat 1,600 calories per day... every day.

   Now, how can that possibly work?

   What if you had a ridiculously active and stressful day and burned far more calories than you usually do. Shouldn't you eat more... especially since you'll be hungrier than usual? And what if you had a very lazy day? Also, depending on your size, you might need to eat less... or more.

   The point is, trying to set your calories with a calculator and a food journal is futile. There is no possible way to know how many you're burning on a daily basis unless you live in a metabolic chamber.

   But just like everything else in our bodies, nature made sure we had very accurate and *instinctive* ways to determine proper food and water ingestion via hunger and thirst, respectively.

   Think about it, if your heart stops beating, you'll die. If you stop breathing, you'll die. And if you stop eating, you'll die. You can be sure that whoever put us on this planet wouldn't make every other physiologic function instinctive and leave something as crucial as nutrition ingestion merely to our intellect.

   Alright, time to discuss the phases of this diet. Onward...

B. The Phases of the Cruise Control Diet

The traditional Cruise Control Diet consists of the following three phases:

1. The Metabolic Reset Phase
2. The Cruise Control Phase
3. The Rapid Fat Burning Phase

Now, I say "traditional" because it can be modified to suit your goals and your lifestyle. And we'll cover that later. But first, let's examine the core program...

The first phase (and arguably the hardest) is somewhat strict. This is where you reset your metabolism by lowering your insulin levels, and hence why I've coined it "The Metabolic Reset Phase". This lasts for two weeks.

The second is called the Cruise Control Phase because your weight loss, and more specifically fat loss, will literally be on cruise control. Here, you're much less strict and this will last for life. If done right (it's very hard to screw it up, trust me) you will never fall of the wagon.

The third is actually an extension of the second and runs together with it. It's also optional but highly recommended. In fact, if you do decide to partake, you'll experience not only rapid fat loss, but a feeling of wellbeing, energy, and strength you haven't felt since your twenties and thirties (perhaps ever). I know that's a big claim, but you really have to experience it to believe it. We'll go over this in detail in chapter IX.

Now, let's discuss the differences between the first two phases. Essentially, they're exactly alike except for cheat meals. In the initial two weeks you're not going to have any sugar besides some fruit. Also, if you're a coffee drinker like myself, feel free to put a little sugar in it. I don't anymore but I did when I started out and I lost weight just fine.

You're doing this in order to lower your insulin levels as much as possible and rebuild your body's natural hunger instinct. You're also training your body to prefer burning fat for energy rather than sugar. Finally, this sugar detox will rid you of most of your cravings. By the time you get into your third week (i.e. phase II) they'll be 75%-80% gone.

This "strict" phase (I'll explain the quotes in a minute) also serves another very important purpose. It will amplify your awareness of the negative effects a heavy carb load has on your body.

Let me explain... carbohydrates are basically sugar and sugar (in large amounts) is very, *very* bad for you. Our bodies were never meant to metabolize sugar... especially not in a non-fibrous form like starch (e.g. pasta, potatoes) and certainly not in the amounts that we're feeding them. We primarily evolved to eat fibrous carbs, namely veggies and some fruit.

I won't go into details here, but if you want to learn just how bad sugar is for your body, there's a great lecture available on YouTube by one of the leading authorities on the subject. His name is Dr. Robert Lustig and he's a pediatric endocrinologist at the University of California San Francisco. Here's the link: **Sugar: The Bitter Truth**.

Now, if you've been carbing up (the way most Americans do) for most of your life, you probably don't feel its negative effects. At least you don't realize them. But you will after you're done with the Metabolic Reset Phase and you have your first cheat meal.

I remember mine vividly. I ate a half a pint of Ben & Jerry's cookie dough ice cream and 20 minutes later I felt like I had been hit by a truck. I passed out at around 9:30 PM – exhausted.

This may sound like an exaggeration but you have to experience it to believe it. Sugar really is that bad for you. Food should give you energy. It shouldn't make you feel prostrated. But that's what sugar and starches unfortunately do.

It's the same thing that happens to a smoker after he quits and relapses several months later. That first cigarette will be nasty. He'll get dizzy, his heart rate will increase, nausea will set in, etc... I know this because I used to smoke... for 15 years! I quit and went back to it several times. And that first cigarette always reminded me how bad smoking really was. Too bad my addiction was stronger than my logic or willpower. But thank God that's finally out of my life.

Getting back to the point... you need to become aware of (on a "visceral level") just how bad sugar really is for you. So even though you'll be cheating in the second phase, eventually... you'll start to loathe cheat meals. I still eat them once a week or so, but mostly dark chocolate, which aside from a little sugar, is very heart healthy.

It's hard to believe how much I don't miss or crave things such as potatoes and bread when I used to eat one or the other with every meal. And you won't miss them either – and that's a good thing.

Now, let's get to the fun part... all the tasty foods you *do* get to eat.

C. Your New Food Pyramid

This eating program is easy to follow and even easier to stick to because aside from sweets, you're only limiting starch from your diet. So all of your meals will revolve around foods you're already eating: meat (e.g. chicken, beef, pork, and wild game), fish, eggs, vegetables, fruits, and nuts.

There are several tasty recipes in your accompanying cookbook, plus I'll be sending you new ones on a regular basis so you never get bored. With that said, let's go over your typical eating day.

The most difficult of all will be breakfast. Why? Because almost all breakfasts are carb and starch heavy (cereal, pancakes, bagels, etc.). Personally, I used to be a big cereal eater before I started this program.

Now, when I eat breakfast (explained below), it's usually a four-egg omelet and 4-5 strips of bacon. Contrary to the *still* widely held belief – despite studies that prove otherwise – eggs are not bad for you and they will not raise your cholesterol (I'll discuss this in depth in the next chapter).

However, and as we'll go over later – **make sure that if you eat bacon or sausages (or any other meat that's typically processed, i.e. lunch/deli meats and cold cuts) that it's uncured and does not contain added nitrates or nitrites or any other chemical preservative.**

The latter are why these meats are harmful to your health (not the fat). You can find this type of bacon in stores such as Whole Foods, Trader Joe's, or even a good butcher shop. Furthermore, Boars Head is a good brand of nitrate-free cold cuts (you'll also find more with a simple Google search, "nitrate free cold cuts).

Now, back to breakfast. To be honest, I don't always eat it. I'm simply not hungry. I've got plenty of food to work on from the night before. So, I drink coffee up until lunchtime, which is around 12-1 PM for me. The bottom line is: whether or not you choose to eat breakfast is up to you. And if you do, avoid the typical starches, cereals, and juices. Have an omelet with veggies instead – even some bacon.

With that said, I'd like to discuss another myth. That is, about breakfast being the most important meal of the day. In short, it's not. Sure, studies have shown that people who skip breakfast are more likely to be overweight than those who don't. However, as scientists say, "correlation does not prove causation".

In other words, these people aren't heavier than their breakfast eating counterparts because they choose to skip breakfast. It's because they eat the wrong foods throughout the rest of the day.

You see, because the whole, "breakfast is the most important meal of the day" myth is so prevalent, health conscious people naturally tend to follow the advice. But those same health conscious people will also eat better than the "skippers" (and perhaps exercise more). So, the fact that they weigh less is because they have better eating habits overall – not because they eat breakfast.

Again, learn to listen to your body. If you're hungry eat. If you're not, don't.

Now, lunch and dinner are basically similar. You should eat a piece of meat or fish with a salad or broccoli, cauliflower, or any other vegetable.

If you're a "meat and potatoes guy" (or gal) the way I used to be, this will feel "funny" at first. And by funny I mean that you won't quite feel satisfied when you've finished your meal. You'll be full – but not satisfied – especially during the first phase, the Metabolic Reset. A good way to counter this is to eat some nuts such as almonds or hazelnuts after your meal. They'll make you feel full *real* fast.

Now, I won't lie... you will miss your starches. By the third week, however, it won't be an issue. Furthermore, you'll see that when you finish eating, you'll feel light and energetic. You won't have that heavy, tired, and sleepy feeling that typically comes on 10-20 minutes after a carb-heavy meal.

You'll understand what I mean when you get into the 2nd phase and you decide to eat some pasta for a cheat meal (discussed shortly).

OK, what about quantities?

Here's the beauty of the program. Eat as much as you want. Now, during your first few days you might go a bit overboard. But don't worry. This will quickly correct itself. Your body will find a balance as long as you're feeding it what it wants and reducing your levels of insulin.

And meal frequency?

As mentioned in the previous section, this is up to you. Whether you eat 3 times a day or 6... or something in between doesn't matter one bit. Just eat when you're hungry.

Like I mentioned before, I'll eat 2-3 times/day and on some days I'll eat a snack when I feel like it. This is always some kind of nut unless I'm craving a cheat meal such as chocolate.

Now, about those cheat meals...

When you enter Phase II, you should eat 1-2 cheat meals per week. Furthermore, you should **eat them without guilt**. Also, don't worry about the quantity. If you want to eat a whole pizza, go ahead. A pint of ice cream? Fine. Whatever your heart desires.

Now, just like in the first few days of the program (where you might overshoot your calories)... you're likely to do the same with your cheat meals. But don't worry – this too will correct itself and you'll find your way. Plus, after a few months you won't feel the need to cheat as much.

One word of caution, however... **I do not advise you to skip your cheat meals if you want them – ever.** What I mean is, don't purposely skip them in order to lose weight faster. You'll only feel deprived. This will make you miserable and you'll feel like you're dieting. You don't want to be dieting, per say. You want to be making better food choices... choices you can stick to for life.

Not to mention, going overboard on your calories for a day can have beneficial effects aside from the psychological ones. You see, when you're losing fat your levels of the hormone leptin also go down. Leptin is a key regulator of fat loss. And when it gets too low it becomes harder to lose weight. By overfeeding once in a while, you essentially shoot it up again so you don't hit plateaus.

Isn't this program great?

What should you drink?

Water or unsweetened ice tea. Ditch the soda (even the diet, calorie-free one; it's loaded with aspartame which is *very bad* for your health). Fruit juice is no good either. It has way too much sugar. For example, when you drink a glass of orange juice you're essentially taking in 3-4 oranges in one shot... without the fiber. You'd never do that if you were eating the fruit whole. Plus, many juices contain additional sweeteners that are bad for you. So again, water or unsweetened ice tea.

A final note on water... another commonly held belief is that you have to drink 8, 8 oz. glasses per day to speed up weight loss. This is ridiculous. First of all, the person who gave us the idea of 8 glasses of water was misquoted. Essentially he said that we should consume about 8, 8 oz. glasses of water per day... *most of which we get from food.*

Just like hunger, your natural sense of thirst will let you know how much you need to drink. Some days, you'll need more. Some days you'll need less. It all comes down to your level of activity and how much you've lost through sweat.

What about alcohol?

I drink once in a while (sometimes, more than I should). However, I stopped drinking beer. Why? Far too many carbs. It's akin to downing liquid bread. Stick to wine and spirits. No fruity cocktails like Margaritas or other sugar-loaded drinks.

Now, a word of advice on alcohol... It makes you hungry because it lowers your blood sugar. This can cause you to go into an eating binge – especially if it's one of those weekend outings with friends (ask me how I know).

With this in mind, if you like to drink you should reserve one of your cheat meals for the nights you go out. And if you go overboard and binge really bad – don't worry. Do not feel guilty either. Life should be enjoyed. Furthermore, if you're eating clean 90% of the time (which you will be because you're limiting your cheat meals to 1-2 times per week) this won't stall your progress much, if at all.

OK, we discussed meats, fish, veggies, and nuts. **But what about fruit?**

Fruit is an amazing food due to its high antioxidant content. However, it is loaded with sugar. Therefore, I don't recommend eating several servings per day. I typically eat a Granny Smith apple a day or some berries (blueberries, blackberries, strawberries, etc...). Additionally, stay away from dried fruits like raisins – far too high in sugar. If you like eating them, do so as part of a cheat meal.

Alright, let's move on to **dairy products**...

As a general rule of thumb, these should be limited. They cause a much larger insulin spike than can be explained by their sugar content (i.e. lactose). Now, if you want to drink a little milk from time to time – it's OK. Just don't go overboard.

I was never big on dairy so this was never an issue for me. I do, however, drink plenty of coffee. Therefore, I add in just a dash of milk to each cup for the "color change". It hasn't affected my weight as far as I can tell. I also put feta cheese in my salads from time to time. It's delicious, and again, never stalled my weight loss nor caused me to gain any of it back. Finally, ice cream is one of my favorite cheat meals.

In the end, it's about finding a balance. While a small amount of dairy might not have a negative impact on *my* waistline, your story might be different. The best bit of advice I can give you here is: experiment. That is, if you'd like to keep dairy products in your diet.

Also, it's important to note that as time goes by, your metabolism will improve dramatically. So, if you're particularly sensitive to dairy today – that might not be the case a couple of months down the road. Again, you'll need to test this out a bit to find your optimal balance.

One final thing as far as dairy is concerned: **do not consume the low-fat versions**. While there is still plenty of debate surrounding this topic, it seems that the fat content of diary blunts the insulin response somewhat. Remember, you want to avoid insulin spikes as much as possible.

Now let's discuss **legumes** such as beans, lentils, and chickpeas...

I used to eat these, *a lot*, but I cut them out entirely. Why? Actually, two reasons... For one, they have a very high carb content. Of course, much of that is soluble fiber. Nevertheless, eating legumes too frequently could affect your weight loss goals. Just like diary, if you're big on these, you'll have to experiment.

Secondly, they're difficult to digest and cause lots of gas. Somehow, that can't be good for you. Based on the laws of nature and evolution, a food that is supposed to be good for us, shouldn't cause us such distress when eating it. That's something you ought to consider.

Always remember: **listen to your body**. If it doesn't feel right after eating a particular food (the way it won't after you eat a big plate of pasta in the second phase of this program) limit it or stay away from it altogether.

Now, before we move on to the next section I'd like to address something that's likely to have crossed your mind. If you're eliminating starches and grains, limiting dairy and legumes, aren't you dramatically increasing your calories from fat... particularly saturated fat?

And the answer is yes, you are. But make no mistake about it: this is a good thing despite what we've been told. For one, saturated fat has gotten a bad rap due to a flawed and biased study (remember the story of Ancel Keys in Chapter II?)

Secondly, you'll be consuming *natural* saturated fat... the kind humans have been eating for millions of years... not the artificial, man-made *trans-fat* which has been proven to cause disease (i.e. the kind found in baked goods, margarine, etc...). And it's no surprise either, our bodies never evolved to eat trans-fats, hence the reason we can't metabolize them properly and the resultant damage.

Finally (and as counter-intuitive as it sounds) a high-fat diet is crucial to getting and staying skinny. Why? Because it keeps you full by delaying stomach emptying. For example, on the days where I eat chicken or a low-fat fish such as haddock I tend to get hungrier much sooner than if I had eaten a steak, lamb, or a piece of fatty fish such as swordfish or salmon.

With that said, I fully understand if you're concerned about eating this way. I was too – very much. In fact, I grew up loathing fat because I thought it was so bad for me.

But the truth is, we've been (*and continue to be*) misled about fat for decades. If you do the research you'll discover that the entire case against fat is built on a house of cards... and mostly responsible for our current obesity epidemic. As such, I've devoted Chapter VII to one of the most controversial medical topics of our days: saturated fat, cholesterol, and heart disease.

But before we get to that, let's discuss two important points: how to shop at the supermarket and how to eat when you go out...

D. How to Shop at the Supermarket and What to Eat at Restaurants

If you exclude the occasional cheat meal, this is basically a whole foods diet. In other words, if the food is not found in nature, you don't eat it. This rule of thumb will go a long way to keeping you fit and healthy.

It has been said that you should only shop in the outer isles of supermarket... and I fully agree. That is where you'll find the whole foods – not in the middle isles that contain mostly packaged, processed foods (loaded with salt and sugar) that wreak havoc on your health.

So, on your next trip to the grocery store, stock up on meats, veggies, fruits, fish, and some nuts for snacks (e.g. almonds, walnuts). Those will be the staple of your diet. Again, avoid anything that comes in a package or a box except for spices or some condiments (discussed below).

Also, you should buy organic whenever possible. I know it can be *prohibitively* expensive (especially if you're not used to shopping this way) but it's definitely worth it. Conventionally grown food is not good for your health for reasons we'll get to later. I didn't believe it at first, but after researching the matter in depth, I no longer eat non-organic foods (*for the most part*) and you shouldn't either.

There are plenty of ways to eat the best quality foods without putting too big of a dent in your bank account. Furthermore, even if it *is* somewhat more expensive, consider the following... you're going to pay for it regardless – either at the supermarket or at the doctor's office. However, the latter will be much more expensive plus it will come at the high cost of your health.

With that said, I believe that it is so crucial you understand this subject matter (and you start eating this way) that I've devoted an entire chapter to it which we'll get to later. But for now, just keep the above in mind.

Moving on...

Do not buy junk food when you're doing your weekly shopping – unless it's for your cheat meal of THAT *day*.

Here's why...

If it's in the house, you'll eat it – much more often than you should. Not many people have the willpower to resist cravings. If you feel like cheating, go out and get your meal, and... either eat it at the store (e.g. a restaurant, ice cream parlor) or bring it back home.

Also, make sure you finish it all... or else, throw the rest away. For example, let's say you're eating Doritos. You'd be wise not to buy a giant bag. But sometimes, your "eyes are bigger than your stomach". So, if you make this mistake and don't finish the entire bag... *throw the rest away*! And as much as I hate wasting food (and consequently, money) I believe it's better to do so rather than damage your health.

OK, now I'd like to take a minute to discuss condiments and dressings. Generally, these are a huge source of hidden sugar... especially those low-fat salad dressings. They're disguised as healthy with their low-fat labels but in truth they're nothing but junk food.

You see, anything that has its natural fat content removed will taste like cardboard if sugar isn't added. Of course, nobody will buy it so the manufacturers add sugar to improve the taste. So, if you're going to buy a salad dressing, choose the full fat version over the low fat one... and above all **learn to read labels**.

However, as you'll see in your accompanying cookbook, you don't really need to buy salad dressing. Extra virgin olive oil, red vinegar, balsamic, or lemon (depending on the vegetable) are all you really need to spice up your veggies and make them really tasty.

As for condiments, these are just as dangerous. For example, ketchup is loaded with sugar and barbecue sauce is even worse. The latter was a bit hard for me to give up. But knowing the damage it causes my body has made it much easier.

Alright... let's move on to restaurants. Is it possible to still eat out on this plan? Of course! It's actually not that hard in most places. Unless you're having a cheat meal, you still follow the same guidelines (i.e. meat/fish and a veggie).

For example, let's say you went to a burger joint. You can still order your bacon cheeseburger. Just have them hold the bun and substitute the French fries for a salad with an oil and vinegar dressing. Of course, it's not as tasty or exciting as eating it the traditional way. So, perhaps you want to save your cheat meals for outings.

A final word regarding this: **don't go overboard with the "rules"**. For instance, let's say you had some pretty strong cravings during the week and you ate a bag of chips on Monday and some cookies on Thursday. Now it's Saturday night and you find yourself in an Italian restaurant. And... for some reason they have nothing but pasta (not a likely scenario but bear with me nonetheless). But... you've already had your two cheat meals for the week.

What should you do?

Easy: eat like everyone else around you. Don't worry about "falling off the wagon" or about controlling your portions or anything of that sort. Enjoy your meal and don't feel guilty about it for a single second.

Sure, this program requires you to exercise a bit of restraint. But you never want to get to the point where you resent the idea of eating healthy. It's counterproductive and will eventually cause you to crack and go back to your old eating habits.

Plus... don't forget that as your metabolism speeds up due to your new diet, these foods won't have as much of a negative impact as they otherwise would. But again, don't use this fact as an excuse to binge more often. As with everything else in life, balance is the key. Finally, you'll understand exactly why this is so important when we go over the chapter on mindset.

E. Your Quick Reference Guide to Good Eating

Eat on a daily basis	Avoid except for cheat meals	Eliminate entirely (except for cheat meals)	Snacks
• Vegetables • Any type of meat (e.g. beef, chicken, turkey, pork, wild game) • Organs (e.g. liver) • Fish • Eggs • Fruit (in moderation; stick to low GI fruit)	• Bread • Potatoes • Pasta • Rice • Beans • Beets • Corn	• Soda (Regular and diet; choose regular over diet due to aspartame) • Fruit juices • Dried fruit • Candy • Pastries • Cookies • Potato chips • Anything that comes prepackaged (e.g. TV dinners)	• Nuts (e.g. almonds, walnuts, hazelnuts) • Uncured ham and other deli cuts • Pickles • Smoked salmon • Roasted peppers

F. One Size Does <u>Not</u> Fit All – Modifying the CCD to Suit Your Lifestyle and Dietary Goals

Personally, I find this the easiest diet to be on. That's because it's not a diet – it's a lifestyle. Of course, not everyone who's tried it feels that way. As such, in the four years or so that I've made this program public, I've worked with a number of people to modify it to their liking. And I'm going to lay out some of these modifications right here.

But before I do, allow me to say this: just like with everything else in life you only get out of it what you put into it. The plan I've proposed requires some sacrifice in order for you to reach your health and fitness goals. However, unlike most other diets, it doesn't require suffering.

You now know how to eat in order to:

a. Lose weight fast.

b. Do so without hunger and cravings.

c. Plus, you can indulge from time to time without stalling your progress.

Again, you're sacrificing but not suffering. However, as mentioned above, not everyone feels that way. Case in point, I had a woman contact me recently to complain this diet wasn't for her. She told me that she couldn't eat only 2 cheat meals per week and was going back to Weight Watchers. I tried to talk her out of it but her mind was made up. So, I wished her well. Of course, I thought she was making a terrible mistake and I've explained why in the initial chapters of this book. But, to each his own (or in this case, her own).

So, where am I going with all of this?

The more you deviate from the core program, the longer it will take you to lose the weight. Furthermore, you won't experience the full range of health benefits you otherwise would. But it all comes down to a balance: what are you willing to give up in order to gain?

In the case of the woman mentioned above, she wasn't willing to give up very much. Obviously this program isn't for her. On the other hand, you can still get great results even if you don't follow my advice to the T. With that said, let me break things down for you in order of importance.

Now, it goes without saying that candy, cakes, and sweets can't be eaten on a daily basis (even in small quantities). If you can't live by this rule then, no offense, but... you'll have to join that woman at Weight Watchers.

Aside from that...

1. **Liquid sugar is enemy #1.** If you drink a lot of juice, soda, energy drinks, or fancy coffees from Starbucks, DD's, or similar stores, and... you switch to water, while doing nothing more, you'll go on to experience a good amount of weight loss.

   In other words, you can still eat bread, potatoes, rice, ketchup, etc. and still shed the pounds. Now, I don't recommend this be the only change you make, but it's far better than any diet plan that includes lots of sugary drinks.

   If you absolutely MUST drink something other than water, here are my suggestions (in order of best to worst):

   i.   Unsweetened ice tea.

   ii. Sweetened ice tea (boil some tea, cool it down, and add a teaspoon of sugar – or better still - Stevia).

   iii. Sweetened homemade lemonade (squeeze 1 lemon in a glass of water and add a teaspoon of sugar or Stevia to it).

   iv. Diet soda – I'm not too happy about listing this here, but with it being as popular as it is, I feel compelled to give you the option. With that said, I'd choose a spoon of sugar over aspartame (the sweetener in diet drinks) any day of the week.

   And if you want to know why, have a look through the following resource (it's very eye-opening): http://aspartame.mercola.com.

2. **Smoothies are enemy #2.** There is absolutely no reason for you to be consuming such large amounts of liquid fruit. It's a sugar bomb of the worst kind: fructose. Aside from ballooning your waistline, fructose is quickly becoming associated with many diseases and health problems (e.g. gout, fatty liver, elevated triglycerides, etc.).

   Eat your fruit whole. And even then, eat it in moderation. And if you really want to go above and beyond as far as fruit is concerned, find out how much your body can tolerate. Everyone's different in this respect and your levels of uric acid (which fructose raises) will let you know where you stand. You can get this simple test performed by requesting it from your doctor. If you're a man, you should aim for 4.0 mg/dL and if you're a woman, 3.5 mg/dL.

3. **Certain condiments are enemy #3.** For example, ketchup, BBQ sauce, and low-fat salad dressings. You can replace the latter with olive oil and vinegar or choose the full-fat version. As for ketchup and BBQ

sauce, if you must eat them, eat them in small quantities and try to slowly phase them out.

4. **Refined carbs are enemy #4** (e.g. white bread, white rice, white pasta, etc.). Not nearly as bad as the above two, but keeping these out of your diet will make weight loss faster and easier.

5. **Potatoes are enemy #5.** I love potatoes. They're probably one of the hardest things I had to give up. Again, they're not nearly as bad as the above, but the fact that they're typically consumed in such large quantities really inhibits losing weight.

   Now, if this is one of the foods you absolutely can't live without, perhaps you can switch to sweet potatoes. They're better for you and less obesogenic. But still, even if you continue to eat white potatoes and severely limit all of the above, you'll be in good enough shape.

6. **Everything else is a mixed bag**: whole grains, dairy, legumes, etc... If those are things you must have on a daily or frequent basis, experiment with them.

So, let me give you an example. I had a gentleman do quite well on the CCD even though he tailored it to his personal preferences. He ate a slice of toast for breakfast every day (I don't remember what else he had but it wasn't cereal, pancakes, or bagels – most likely eggs). Also, he couldn't drink only water so he made his own sweetened lemonade.

In short, he changed the rules a bit to suit his personal preferences but followed the program overall (i.e. eliminated most starches, stopped drinking sodas, and stuck to 1 cheat meal per week). And, he went on to lose the weight quite easily.

Could he have lost it easier and faster? For sure, but it would have required a bigger sacrifice than he was willing to make. And that's completely understandable. In the end, only you can decide what you're willing and not willing to give up to get what you want.

Alright, now before we wrap this up, let me leave you with the following bit of advice: do not modify the first phase of the program. I insist you follow the rules to the T in the first couple of weeks. It is the only way to experience a rapid drop in your insulin levels and your weight.

This is important because, getting a great start will keep you going – wanting to get fitter and healthier. Additionally, it will help you give up some of the things you might be thinking are impossible to live without. If you can purge yourself of the toxins entirely – you'll really feel their negative effects on your body once you eat them again. This might be enough to make you shun them altogether.

So, that wraps it up for modifications. Stay on track as much as possible and you won't be disappointed. On the same token, don't drastically alter your life if those changes aren't ones you can live with long-term. It will only lead to failure down the road. Find your balance and stick to it.

Alright, let's move on to one of the most controversial topics in public health...

VII. The Shocking Truth About Cholesterol and Saturated Fat

As you read about in Chapter II, the whole crusade against saturated fat started back in the 50's with Ancel Keys' 7-country study. And if you remember, he deliberately manipulated his results to *falsely* prove his point (i.e. that consuming too much saturated fat in your diet leads to heart disease). Of course, when you take this into consideration, it's obvious that saturated fat has no bearing on heart disease.

Nevertheless, several studies have been conducted since. And after all these years, the medical establishment *still* hasn't been able to show that saturated fat is to blame for our ills. In fact, saturated fat can't be blamed for anything... other than raising heart-protective HDL (or "good" cholesterol; more on this later).

But don't just take my word for it... a huge meta-analysis was published in the prestigious *American Journal of Clinical Nutrition* in 2010 demonstrating this fact. By the way, a meta-analysis is when researchers combine the results of several similar studies in order to determine correlation with a much smaller probability of error due to the higher number of control subjects.

Getting back to the point... this study, titled "Meta-analysis of prospective cohort studies evaluating the association of saturated fat with cardiovascular disease" concluded the following:

> A meta-analysis of prospective epidemiologic studies showed that **there is no significant evidence for concluding that dietary saturated fat is associated with an increased risk of CHD* or CVD*.** More data are needed to elucidate whether CVD risks are likely to be influenced by the specific nutrients used to replace saturated fat.

*CDH: Coronary Heart Disease; CVD: Cardiovascular Disease.

Furthermore, this meta-analysis was huge, including 21 studies and 347,747 subjects followed over 5-23 years. And this is just *one* study proving that saturated fat is harmless. There are several others. All it takes is a few simple searches on Google to discover the mountains of information available on this topic.

Why this study never made the front page of all newspapers, Time Magazine, and became the featured story of every nightly news channel is beyond me. Perhaps, it's just too much all at once given the fact that we've been fed the low-fat dogma for decades. Still, these findings are slowly seeping into the mainstream media. The public is starting to wake up.

Nevertheless, it will take some time before these results (and proper recommendations) are universally embraced. But trust me, we're going to look back 20-30 years from now and laugh at the traditional low-fat advice. Actually, the laughter will more likely be tears, considering the amount of devastation it has caused to millions of people worldwide. It's almost as ludicrous as when doctors used to smoke and endorse specific brands in paid advertisements.

Now let's look at an equally controversial subject: **cholesterol**...

First off, it doesn't matter how much cholesterol you eat in your diet. Here's why: your liver is responsible for making approximately 75%-80% of the cholesterol found in your blood. The rest comes from your diet. And if you eat foods high in cholesterol, your liver compensates for this by producing less.

Now, about 30% of the population are known as "hyper-responders". That is, eating foods high in cholesterol produces a corresponding increase in their blood. However, this increase is of the good, "fluffy" kind that is actually protective against heart disease due to its anti-oxidant properties. This will all make sense in a minute, but for now... know this...

There is no such thing as bad cholesterol!

I know what you're thinking, however, the above really is not a misprint. But what about LDL, you ask? Here's the scoop...

Cholesterol is just cholesterol. It is a waxy substance that isn't soluble in blood. Therefore, in order to be transported to areas where it is needed (yes, you need cholesterol to stay alive) it has to be bundled with proteins – lipoproteins to be exact.

LDL (or low density lipoprotein) transports it to your organs. And HDL (or high density lipoprotein) takes it back to your liver for recycling. What doctors, nutritionists, and basically everyone else refers to as bad cholesterol is just cholesterol packed inside LDL.

Now, while there is no good or bad cholesterol, **there is good LDL and bad LDL.** It comes in two patterns. Pattern A is large and fluffy (what we discussed above). It is considered harmless and may even offer protection against heart disease. Pattern B is small and dense. This is the stuff that clogs your arteries and can lead to heart attacks and strokes.

Here's why this information is crucial – and perhaps lifesaving: **you can have perfectly normal cholesterol levels and still have a heart attack!** In fact...

> A nationwide study conducted by UCLA School of Medicine found that 75 percent of patients hospitalized for a heart attack had LDL cholesterol within the so-called safe range - below 130 mg/dl. (21 percent of the patients were taking a statin cholesterol-lowering drug.)
>
> Even more astounding, 50 percent of patients had LDL less than 100 mg/dL - considered optimal levels! The mean LDL cholesterol among the hospitalized patients was 104.9 mg/dL.

In other words, you could have "optimal" cholesterol because of a statin, feel safe with your "healthy" levels, and then... as you're strolling down the street one day... drop to your knees with crushing chest pain and die before the paramedics arrive at the scene.

And even though this scenario happens daily, I'm *not* saying this to scare you. In fact, by knowing this information you can take the next steps to find out where you stand and correct any problems that exist. Then, you can really rest easy knowing that a heart attack is not likely in your future.

So, how can you know if your LDL is made up of the deadly pattern B or the safe – even healthy – pattern A?

All it takes is a simple blood test. It's known as the Vertical Auto Profile or the VAP test. Now, a word of warning: your doctor may try to talk you out of it if you're not at high risk for heart disease. Regardless, **insist on getting tested**. After all, this is your life we're talking about!

Furthermore, here are two more reasons to get a VAP test:

1. So you can measure the improvement in your health as you progress through this diet. Try to get tested before you start and then 3 months later. The results will be shocking (in a good way).

2. The conventional cholesterol test uses derived methods to calculate LDL from your triglycerides (hence the reason you're required to fast for about 12 hours before getting tested).

   People on a low-carb diet have very low triglycerides compared to the average population (that's good). However, this causes your LDL levels to measure higher than they truly are. In contrast the

VAP is a direct cholesterol measurement and will give you the more extensive and accurate numbers. Furthermore, you don't need to fast before taking it.

And one more thing regarding the VAP... don't be surprised if you doctor has never heard it (mine hadn't). Surprisingly, many physicians *still* aren't up to date on the latest cholesterol screening techniques. In any case, it won't hurt to print a few pages from the test's official website and have them with you at your next doctor's visit.

OK, so what should you do if your test comes back pattern B? Nothing - because by following The Cruise Control Diet you'll naturally revert to pattern A. Simply take the test again in 3 months to track your improvement.

Now, let's discuss an equally important topic regarding cholesterol: HDL.

Unlike LDL, levels of HDL are directly correlated with heart disease. More specifically, the lower your HDL, the higher your chances of having a heart attack. On the contrary, higher levels (especially over 60) are extremely protective against cardiac events.

But here's the problem...

Raising your HDL to 60 and over is nearly impossible (if you follow conventional advice, that is). The typical recommendations are exercise and moderate alcohol consumption (e.g. 1-2 glasses of wine/day). And while both of these help, their effect is very modest.

The other commonly prescribed option is niacin or vitamin B3. And while it *has* been shown to raise HDL by 15%-35%, many people can't tolerate its side effects (namely, flushing). Furthermore, the increase in HDL as a result of niacin doesn't seem to offer the same protection against heart disease than if it was raised naturally.

In fact, a recent study of 3,414 patients (the AIM-HIGH trial) was stopped early because those participants taking a statin plus niacin experienced a higher number of strokes than those just taking statins.

So, what's the secret to naturally raising HDL?

As hard as it is to believe, **the best way to send HDL soaring is to eat saturated fat.** Now, bear with me for a moment while I explain why this is the case...

Unfortunately, when doctors caution against eating saturated fat, they lump every kind together. But the fact is, not all saturated fat is created equal. There's a good kind and a *very bad* kind.

Trans-fat is a perfect example of the latter. It's a man-made substance used in foods such as such baked goods to preserve their shelf life. But here's the problem with that: it's not found in nature and thus our bodies were never made to metabolize it. The result? It creates inflammation, sends your bad LDL through the roof, slashes your HDL, and eventually "clogs your arteries".

On the contrary, good saturated fat such as the kind found in grass-fed beef is loaded with heart protective omega-3's (like in fish). And while this type of fat may increase your LDL to a small degree, the increase is primarily the good, pattern A LDL. Furthermore, since it also increases your HDL it maintains a safe LDL/HDL ratio.

Which brings us to the next point: **which cholesterol numbers really matter?** New research has shown that it's not enough to look at HDL and LDL (or even total cholesterol) in isolation. In order to get a better picture of heart disease risk we have to examine the ratio of one to the other.

For example...

- You should aim for an HDL/Total cholesterol ratio of 0.24 and above.

- Your triglycerides should be no more than twice your level of HDL. And by the way, if you've never had an advanced cholesterol-screening test like the VAP, this ratio can be used to determine if you're making healthy pattern A LDL or deadly pattern B. A ratio of greater than 2 (triglycerides / HDL) indicates the latter.

- An HDL/LDL ratio of 0.3 is desirable while 0.4 and above is ideal.

However, in order to get those ratios *without drugs* you have to feed your body the right foods. And as mentioned above, if your numbers are off, you're simply not eating right.

Know this: **whatever makes you fat also makes you sick**. And if you're currently overweight and your cholesterol is off, you're getting too many carbs and sugars in your diet. Furthermore, your insulin levels are too high causing your cholesterol to soar. The only way to reverse this trend is to lower the carb content of your diet.

I think we've covered this topic in enough detail. But if you'd like to learn more (I actually encourage you to) you should have a read through the book titled, "**The Great Cholesterol Con**" by Dr. Michael Kendrick.

Now, before we wrap up this chapter I'd like to leave you with the following in order to drive the above points home...

Cholesterol is your friend – not your enemy. It makes up to 50% of every cell membrane in your body and 12-13% of your entire brain. Reducing it to artificially low levels via drugs is not desirable and comes with many side effects (e.g. memory loss, muscle damage).

I know that many have hailed statins as "the aspirin of the 20th century". However, these same people will be singing a different tune when the class action lawsuits start snowballing because of the onset of delayed (and life-threatening) side effects).

As for heart disease? It is increasingly becoming more accepted that inflammation is the major culprit. Cholesterol is just an innocent party (almost). Here's what I mean by that...

Let's say you consume a diet high in sugars, processed foods, and... on top of this – you smoke a pack of cigarettes a day. You're essentially creating inflammation throughout your body. When this is happening in your arteries, it forms what is known as "plaques". So, cholesterol is sent to that area to do its job: repair the damage (think of it as "spackle").

Now, in order to repair the damage, you need to create new cells. And as we discussed above, 50% of your cells' membranes are made of cholesterol. Therefore, when you have inflammation in your body, you'll have higher cholesterol. This is a normal healing response.

But here's the major problem, based on the above hypothetical diet, your LDL would most likely be small, dense pattern B. Therefore, it would get stuck between your arteries' cell lining. If it gets stuck, it won't circulate. And anything that doesn't circulate gets oxidized or becomes rancid.

This creates a vicious circle further amplifying the inflammatory response, increasing the size of the plaque, and eventually narrowing your arteries down to the point where you have a heart attack or stroke (it's a little more complicated than that, but this is the basic concept).

Now, when surgeons (or pathologists during autopsies) examine the insides of arteries, they notice these plaques are filled with fatty deposits and cholesterol. Based on this, many assume that it's the cholesterol causing the problem... where in reality it's the reverse. The cholesterol is essentially the symptom of the disease. The cause is inflammation.

If you're concerned about heart disease and cholesterol and would like to learn more, I also recommend you read **The Great Cholesterol Lie** by Dr. Dwight Lundell.

OK, enough about cholesterol. Let's switch gears now to a topic that few people like to talk about: exercise...

VIII. Exercise: Do You Even Need It to Lose Weight?

This will probably come as a surprise but exercise is *not* a great way to lose weight. I know that this goes against everything you've been told – more so than anything else in this book – but it's true.

And studies prove it...

In fact, a 2009 article in Time Magazine titled, *"Why Exercise Won't Make You Thin"* went on to explain the reason based on the results published in the peer-reviewed journal PLos ONE by Dr. Timothy Church.

Specifically...

> *"Church's team randomly assigned into four groups 464 overweight women who didn't regularly exercise. Women in three of the groups were asked to work out with a personal trainer for 72 min., 136 min., and 194 min. per week, respectively, for six months. Women in the fourth cluster, the control group, were told to maintain their usual physical-activity routines. All the women were asked not to change their dietary habits and to fill out monthly medical-symptom questionnaires.*
>
> *The findings were surprising. **On average, the women in all the groups, even the control group, lost weight, but the women who exercised — sweating it out with a trainer several days a week for six months — did not lose significantly more weight than the control subjects did.** (The control-group women may have lost weight because they were filling out those regular health forms, which may have prompted them to consume fewer doughnuts.) **Some of the women in each of the four groups actually gained weight, some more than 10 lb. each."***

Now, why do you suppose that happened?

Well... like diet, the typical advice on this part of the equation is loaded with myths and misconceptions. For example, here's a popular one: you have to spend several hours per week in the gym doing chronic cardio (i.e. sweating like a pig on the treadmill) if you want to burn off your belly fat.

But nothing could be further from the truth. In fact, **the majority of your weight loss (as much as 80%) is directly due to your diet**. In other words, exercise is much less important than you think when it comes to losing weight. Furthermore, the type of exercise most often recommended for weight loss will do the exact opposite. Here's why...

For most of us, working out isn't fun. It's something we simply believe we *must* do to get slim and stay healthy. After all, that's what the "experts" have told us, so it must be true, right?

With that said, if you happen to exercise, chances are you consider it a chore – a "necessary evil" if you will. And because you don't enjoy it (even though it's good for you) you reward yourself for doing it.

Unfortunately, that reward typically takes the form of a calorie bomb – the big bacon cheeseburger and fries, the huge all-topping pizza, that nice piece of chocolate cake, etc. etc... You know, all of the things that make us fat and make the problem worse.

And here's the tragedy of it all...

Exercise burns a lot less calories than you think. On the flipside, it builds up a massive appetite... that, and a sense of entitlement (i.e. I "deserve" to eat junk food because I'm burning it off). In the end, you end up eating many more calories than you burned off.

And the kicker?

They're the worst type of calories. The final result is to become fatter (and ultimately sicker) than if you didn't exercise at all.

Did you know that you're already getting the best type of exercise you can possibly get... you're just not getting enough of it? What's that you ask? **Walking**: it's the healthiest form of physical activity and you should do it as often as possible.

And here's the best part... you don't have to "schedule" it into your life. Sure, you can set a certain time during the day to walk (e.g. first thing in the morning) and that's fine.

However when you get the diet part of the equation right – everything else will become automatic. As you'll soon discover, your body will strive to maintain perfect "energy balance". It will move as much or as little as it has to in order to maintain its desired weight.

In other words, you will want to move because you'll have loads more energy. Not to mention, if you're overweight, your fat cells will start releasing fatty acids into your blood stream that will need to be burned off. Therefore, you'll move whether you like it or not.

By the way... this might sound a bit far fetched, but trust me, in a few weeks from today, that's what's going to happen and you're going to love it.

With that said... it's always a good idea to have a little motivation. And nothing will motivate you to walk more than a pedometer. **Get and always carry one in your pocket or purse**.

Alright, now even though exercise isn't the best way to lose weight – you should still strive to get some in. Mind you, it's not necessary to lose weight, but it does have amazing health benefits. Furthermore, it does aid weight loss in a different way: it makes your muscles more sensitive to insulin. Therefore, you'll need to secrete less during your meals, and thus, won't store fat as readily.

The best type of exercise you can do (aside from walking) is some form of resistance training. This could be weight training, bodyweight exercises, kettle bell workouts, etc...

OK, that wraps it up as far as exercise is concerned. Now, it's time to go over one of the most advanced strategies for losing weight: phase III of The Cruise Control Diet (warning: not for the faint of heart!)

IX. Phase III: It's Time to Put Your Fat Loss on "Steroids"

If you follow the simple plan outlined in this book, you WILL lose all your extra body fat – both quickly and easily. However, there is an advanced strategy you can work into the plan that will get those pounds off even faster. Not only that, it will make you feel more alert, much more energetic, it will virtually eliminate any cravings you have left, and in general give you a sense of wellbeing you haven't felt in years (perhaps ever).

But before I get into the details, I'd like to make the following points clear...

1. **You should *not* start using this strategy until you've been on the CCD for at least a month.**

   Why?

   Because, your cells might be too insulin resistant if you've been eating a carb-heavy diet up until now. Your body needs some time to lower this resistance and this is crucial to making the strategy work.

2. This strategy is not required – at all – to get to your goal weight. You'll do just fine without it. However, it will get you there faster. Plus... if you'd like to go *beyond* your goal weight and become super-lean (I'm talking about six-pack abs) this is the way to do it.

So, what's this strategy I speak of?

It's called intermittent fasting (or IF) because you do exactly that... fast for short periods of time. The fast can last as little as 16 hours or as long as 24. It is not recommended that you fast longer than that because the majority of the benefits of this method are mostly realized in those first 24 hours.

Now, this might sound difficult to do, but I assure you it's very, very easy. Remember, as a fat burner you won't experience hunger the same you do as a sugar burner (again, why I recommend you don't start this for at least a month into your diet). It will come on much slower and without any of the weakness and "jitteriness".

In fact, I've gotten to the point where I can go lift weights after not eating for 16-17 hours without any problems. Prior to this diet, if I didn't eat 1-2 hours before I went to the gym I wouldn't have enough energy to finish the workout.

Alright, let's go over some typical examples of IF...

There's the 16-18 hour fast. This is the one I do on a daily basis. I'll eat dinner around 8PM, and... I won't eat again until 12-1PM the next day. In a sense, I'm just skipping breakfast – it's simple and it works. My body fat sits at 10-11% and dropping (very slowly at this point but dropping nonetheless). Not to mention, my abs are actually showing for the first time in my life and I do ZERO cardio or even situps.

Then there's the longer 24 hour fast. Here you would basically go from dinner to dinner or lunch to lunch without eating anything in between. For example, you'd eat your dinner at 8PM on Sunday night and then not eat again until Monday at 8PM.

Unlike the 16-hour fast, this is a little more challenging because you're awake for more hours before you eat. Furthermore, you shouldn't do this more than once or twice per week.

Others follow something called the "Warrior Diet" where essentially you eat all of your food within a 4-5 hour window (e.g. between 12PM-4PM every day).

Now, if this is the first time you've heard of IF, it probably sounds insane to you. Why would anyone in his or her right mind do such a thing?

That's exactly what I thought when I first came across this strategy... that is, until I researched it a bit further. You see, scientists are discovering that IF actually has a range of anti-aging and other benefits. The general consensus is that eating is a stressor for your body. And by eating less (i.e. calorie restriction) you're putting less strain on your system.

IF has also been shown to:

1. Increase Growth Hormone (GH). This is a primary fat-burning and muscle-building hormone with strong anti-aging properties (ever hear of Hollywood celebrities that pay $1,000's for GH injections? Well, you don't need to do anything of the sort. IF has been shown to increase your GH by up to 600%!)

2. Lower insulin levels and increase your cells' insulin sensitivity (i.e. the exact effect you're aiming for by following this low-starch, low-sugar diet).

3. Increase lipolysis and fat oxidation. In other words, your body releases your stored fat into your bloodstream more readily to be burned for energy. This is why (as I mentioned above) I'm able to go lift heavy weights after a 16-17 hour fast without batting an eye.

Finally, in addition to the benefits just listed, IF has another advantage: calorie restriction. So, not only are you eating less (which, along with the proper nutrition, is the key to weight loss) you're also priming your body to make better use of the "fuel" you put into it. In essence, it's a dual-action strategy and that's why it works so well to burn off body fat.

With that said, I'm sure a few red flags are going off in your head about this method... especially if it's the first time you've been exposed to it. Well, let me put your mind at ease.

For starters, going without food for this long will not make your metabolism crash. I promise. Remember, our physiology is not that inefficient that we need to eat every 3 hours just to keep our metabolism "stoked". We were meant to go for long periods of time without food or else we would have never risen to the top of the food chain.

However, I'm sure you still have your doubts. And while this field of research is still relatively new, there are several studies proving that IF is in fact, a very healthy approach to eating.

For example...

In a study conducted at the University of Nottingham England, researchers found that when they made 29 men and women fast for 3 days, their metabolic rate did not change. That's a full 72 hours without food!

In another study performed at the Pennington Biomedical Research Center, men and women who fasted every other day for a period of 22 days experienced no decrease in their resting metabolic rate.

And finally, not using fasting, but extreme calorie restriction, a study published in 1999 found that people who were on very low calorie diets and on a resistance exercise program (i.e. weight training) did not see a decrease in resting metabolic rate, and these people were only eating 800 calories a day for 12 weeks.

You can find a lot more information regarding IF by doing a simple Google search. But please note... most of the results will be blogs by men who are using this strategy to get to very low levels of body fat (i.e. that coveted 6-pack abs look).

And while this might not be your cup of tea, IF is not just about getting a 6-pack or becoming extremely lean. The fact is, getting down to single-digit body fat so your abs show is *very* difficult. Those final 10 or so pounds are very difficult to come off. However, IF has made it *almost* easy.

Just imagine how well it will work if you use it fairly early in your weight loss journey... especially since this weight is much easier to take off. So, don't discount this powerful method to get into amazing shape because a bunch of "meat-heads" are primarily using it.

With that said, let me describe it for you in a little more detail. As I mentioned above, I get my last meal in around 8 PM. I wake up in the morning between 6:30-7:00 and head to work. Before I get to the office, I grab myself a cup of coffee with a tiny splash of milk (just to change the color) – absolutely no sugar.

Hunger doesn't even begin to set in until 10:00-10:30 AM – that's 14 to 14.5 hours of fasting. And even then, it's not like any kind of hunger you've experienced before: no weakness or jittery feelings. On the contrary, you're extremely alert. That's the best way I can describe it. You really have to experience it firsthand to understand.

The point is to keep busy for the next couple of hours until it's time for lunch. And when chow time does roll around, you'll enjoy your meal like never before. On top of that, you'll feel a surge of energy if you break your fast with the right foods (i.e. the ones recommended as part of this plan). Again, you have to experience it to truly appreciate what I'm talking about. Words really can't do it justice.

Now, along with the benefits I've just listed, you'll enjoy much faster fat loss. Plus, you'll do so while sparing your lean mass. This will go a long way towards ensuring your metabolism doesn't slow down and you end up on the dreaded plateau.

So, let's recap the basic principles:

1. Abstain from food for at least 16 hours (e.g. eat dinner and then eat lunch the next day).
2. You're allowed to drink water, coffee, or tea during your fast. Don't use more than a splash of milk for the latter, and absolutely no sugar.
3. Break your fast with something healthy.

Now, a word of warning on the last point: do not under any circumstance attempt to fast if you don't know what your next meal will be. In other words, don't head off to work in the fasted state, wait until 12 or 1 PM rolls around, and then start looking for something to eat.

Why?

Because by this point you're going to be hungry – especially during the first few days of starting IF. This hunger can easily overwhelm your willingness to eat clean and you could start downing all kinds of unhealthy foods and snacks. Of course, that defeats the purpose of this method entirely. So, pack a lunch and bring it with you to work, or in general, have food available to you when it's time to eat.

Now, want to make this method even more effective? Get a workout in right before you break your fast. Make this some kind of resistance training (e.g. free weights, kettle bells) or HIIT (e.g. sprints) – no cardio. Then, eat your largest meal right after your workout, and keep the next meal (or meals) smaller.

If you can't work out until later in the day then you have to follow a slightly different protocol. For example, I work out at 5PM on most days of the week. I break my fast around 12-ish with a smaller meal (approximately 35%-40% of my calories; I don't count them – it's just an estimate). Then, I eat a huge meal after my workout around 8ish and I'm good to go until the next day in the afternoon.

Again, this might seem a bit strange if you're used to grazing every few hours. But the benefits you'll enjoy by giving your body ample time without having to break down food (i.e. so it can burn your stored fat) can't be stressed enough.

In short, you just have to try it to understand. Now, let's move on the next section – somewhat of a philosophical one – but crucial to your long-term success...

X. Why Lasting Weight Loss is Really About Mind Over Matter

This short chapter was missing from the first edition, and for a good reason: I had yet to write it. And I hadn't written it because, up until now, I didn't really understand the concept I'm about to reveal to you.

You see, I've been on this program for just over four yearss now. For me, it's not a diet – it's a lifestyle: one that has drastically improved my body composition and overall health. And at this point, I know, deep down inside that I will never have a weight problem again (that is, unless I get struck by severe illness; knock on wood).

My mindset has completely shifted. I'm no longer a dieter trying to lose weight and keep it off like I had been for years. I'm a fit, healthy person. And, **a fit, healthy person doesn't diet and doesn't concern themselves with weight loss** (for the most part). In essence, I've become someone else – someone better – with completely new habits and outlook on health and nutrition.

Now, this doesn't happen overnight but it's absolutely crucial if you're to break the dreaded cycle of yo-yo-ing. The first step is having a sensible plan you can follow which will allow you to reach your goals without suffering. Furthermore, it has to be sustainable. The Cruise Control Diet *is* such a plan.

And if you follow it, again, you *will* shed the weight both faster and easier than you thought possible. Additionally, you'll start to immerse yourself in all different topics surrounding health and nutrition. It's inevitable as you begin to feel better and more energetic. You'll slowly start to transition into that person I described above. And if you can stay in this state long enough (e.g. 6-12 months) you'll eventually become that person: healthy, fit, and fully in control of their weight.

It's only a matter of time. But just imagine it... do you know how amazing you'll feel knowing you're in total control of weight for the first time in years (perhaps, ever)? So, keep these short paragraphs in mind when you hit a stumbling block. Stay patient and work through them because the reward at the end of the tunnel is just too grand to give up on.

Now, a final word regarding those stumbling blocks: they will come. And at times you'll want to jump the gun and try something else – perhaps go back to Weight Watchers or another program that lets you eat "anything you want" provided it's portion controlled and you keep track of calories.

But always remember, this flies in the face of what we just discussed: **a fit, healthy, person doesn't diet and doesn't concern themselves with weight loss**. On the contrary, if you have to rely on counting, tracking, and journaling to stay slim you will always be a dieter – one that's constantly fighting the possibility of relapse. Don't be that person. Again, make the small sacrifice for the ultimate reward.

XI. The Best Money You Can Ever Spend

As you can imagine, food is big business in the US. And like it or not, a business's major motive is profit. It's only logical. However, that doesn't fare too well for you and I when it comes to the things we put in our bodies.

I'm sure you've heard the old adage, "You are what you eat". Well, what do you think happens when you continue to poison yourself with the pesticides, hormones, and other chemicals found in conventionally grown food?

Obviously, you get sick. Maybe not today or tomorrow but down the road in one way or another.

Something to consider...

So, that's one of the main reasons that I have stopped buying conventionally grown food... and why you should too if your health is important to you. And before I get into the details of how much better organic and locally grown food is for your body... let's take a moment to consider two other important benefits:

1. **The ethical treatment of animals**. I love animals and despise cruelty towards them. Unfortunately, the food industry doesn't share the same views.

    They house pigs in tiny cages so they never get to move during their entire (*miserable*) lives. They pump chickens full of hormones so they plump up fast – far faster than their legs can support them – essentially crippling them. Then, they lie around in their own feces and urine and get sick. In turn they get pumped full of antibiotics... which you end up consuming.

    I could go on and on about this. However, there's an amazing documentary called **Food, Inc.** that you should get and watch immediately. Furthermore, you should spread the message.

    If enough of us vote against these practices *with our wallets...* it's possible that one day they might stop.

    Of course, you could stop eating animals altogether the way vegetarians do. However, I don't think that's either practical or even healthy. These animals were put on this Earth for a reason.

    And as much as I hate the thought that the pork chop sitting in my plate was a cute little piglet just a few weeks ago, I still continue to eat it. Why? Because that's its purpose in life. If farm animals weren't part of our food supply there would be no need for them to exist. All livestock would eventually disappear.

Now, I know I'm starting to go off tangent here (*I really do love animals and this is a topic dear to my heart*) so I'll wrap it up with this: **you can still eat animals while respecting their life. Please do so ethically**.

2. **Buying from your local farms and farm stands is one of the best things you can do. For a couple of reasons actually**:

   a. You'll be supporting your local your community and its economy. And what's better than that... especially in these tough economic times?

   b. It is much easier on your wallet than shopping in the organic section of your supermarket.

Now, let's go back to the issue of health. When you shop organic (or even better, from your local farm) you're buying an animal that has been fed its natural diet. Take beef, for example... conventionally raised cows are fed a diet of corn and grains to fatten them up. However, their natural diet is grass and the grains make them sick. As such, they're pumped full of antibiotics and then sold to you.

If you eat diseased food – the same food your body relies on to nourish and repair itself – obviously you'll end up with disease as well. Perhaps not today, or next month, but eventually it all adds up.

Continuing with our beef example, there's also another thing to take into consideration: its saturated fat content. Throughout this book I've told you, over and over again, that saturated fat is not bad for you. However, that's not entirely true. You see, it comes down to the *composition* of that fat. Specifically, its Omega-3 fatty acid to Omega-6 fatty acid ratio.

Without getting into too many details, the ideal ratio of O-3 to O-6 fats in your diet should be close to 1:3, 1:2, even 1:1. However, the typical American diet is closer to 1:15 or even 1:20. This creates inflammation throughout your body. And as we discussed in the chapter on cholesterol, this leads to heart disease and other ailments.

> **SIDENOTE:** This is the reason why fish-oil supplements have become so popular lately (i.e. their anti-inflammatory omega-3 content) and why doctors recommend eating fish at least once per week.

Now, grass fed beef has on O-3 to O-6 ratio of approximately 1:3 while grain fed beef is more like 1:27! In other words, it's highly pro-inflammatory. And so are all the other meats that have been raised conventionally.

With this in mind, you should *only* consume cage-free chickens and beef and pork that have been fed their *natural* diets (i.e. grass and vegetarian feed, respectively).

Additionally, you should avoid all farm-raised fish. They are raised in extremely polluted waters. The fish end up getting sick and pumped full of antibiotics. Finally, you end up putting that disease into your body. Always buy wild caught fish.

Now, while all this sounds good and well... there is a major drawback to eating organic: its prohibitive cost... especially at stores such as Whole Foods. Groceries can cost up to 3 times more than at supermarkets that stock conventionally grown food. It's a tough pill to swallow, no doubt.

However, consider this: you're going to pay whether you choose to buy organic or conventional... either at the supermarket or in medical bills down the road. Something very important to keep mind.

With that said, you can eat the highest quality food and still stay within your weekly budget.

How?

By shopping local. There is a great site (**www.localharvest.org**) where you can locate local farms and farm stands just about anywhere in the US. Sure, it will take a little more of your time than just driving down to your local supermarket... but trust me... it's well worth it. And again, you'll be doing a great service to your local community which will pay off in spades.

And one last thing before we wrap up as far as organic is concerned. Not all local farms will be organic. It's very expensive to become certified by the USDA and not all farms are big enough or have a large enough budget to do so.

However, that doesn't necessarily mean that their food is in any way inferior to the ones that are certified. Also, non-organic farms *may* use antibiotics in certain cases if any animal gets sick whereas organic farms will put it down. Some antibiotic use is fine as long as the animals are being fed their natural diets and are not getting sick because of overcrowding, poor food, or other inhumane living conditions.

The best thing you can do is visit the farms closest to you. Have the owners give you a tour. Then, you can see with your own eyes how the animals are treated and their overall practices.

I really hope this chapter convinced you to buy organic, or better yet, local if you don't already.

XII. The Biggest Weight Loss Breakthrough of Our Times

The first edition of this book was released in January 2012. And a lot has changed since then regarding our understanding of health and nutrition. But nothing has been more groundbreaking than the discovery of how the *microbiome* regulates our weight. As such, this compelled me to release a new edition in order to include this critical chapter.

Here's the scoop...

Right now there are approximately 100 trillion bacteria living inside your intestines. They've been found to control everything from your digestion, to your immune system, your mood, and most of all, your weight. Not only that, they outnumber your human cells by a factor of 10 to 1.

In fact, did you know that with more than 100 trillion bacterial cells to the 10 trillion human cells in your body, you're basically more bacterial than you are human? That's the reason why these little bugs are so important. And anything that upsets their balance may lead to serious consequences.

You see, even though these bacteria are vital to your wellbeing, they're not all friendly. In fact, there's a constant war going on between those that keep you healthy and slim and the ones that make you sick and fat. And when the bad guys win the battle, they start crowding out the good guys and take up more space in your digestive tract. This is known as gut dysbiosis.

At this point, you are essentially at the mercy of these bacteria. They're literally pulling your strings – like puppet masters – to do their bidding. And they are very, *very* manipulative.

So, when you find yourself caving into those cravings for ice cream, candy, or potato chips... knowing full well that you're falling off the wagon and forcing your body to store more belly fat... it may not be your willpower that's at fault.

In fact, according to a recent study at the University of California San Francisco, your microbiome communicates with your brain, telling you what to crave and even changes your taste receptors so you prefer certain foods over others.

According to lead researcher Athena Aktipis:

> *"Microbes have a lot of potential ways to manipulate us into eating or not eating certain foods... so if you have a gut filled*

> *with microbes that depend on sugar... those microbes would then be under strong pressure to get you to eat more of what they depend on, potentially leading to cravings for those foods."*

To make matters worse, they seem to be more efficient at pulling energy from food and turning it into fat... fat that ends up in your belly, thighs, butt, or anyplace else you happen to store it.

Now, according to scientists, a healthy gut contains about 80% good bacteria to 20% bad. Given this, you have to take the proper steps to both reach *and* maintain that ratio.

For starters, avoid the toxins that are like kryptonite for your friendly bugs. These include antibiotics, artificial sweeteners, pesticides, fluoride, and chlorine, to name a few.

SIDENOTE: This is another reason why it's very important to eat locally sourced or even organic food devoid of pesticides and animals that aren't administered antibiotics on a regular basis. You end up ingesting those toxins which go on to cause gut dysbiosis, GI disturbances, and weight gain.

Next, get plenty of fiber. Now, with The Cruise Control Diet, you're covered on that front as you'll be eating lots and lots of vegetables. That said, one of the best sources of fiber is the Granny Smith Apple.

In fact, Washington State University researchers demonstrated that the fiber of these green apples escapes digestion by your stomach acids and ends up in your colon unscathed. Once there, the good bacteria ferment it, producing a substance known as butyrate. And butyrate acts like a fertilizer for the friendly bugs.

And finally, **make sure to supplement with a quality probiotic**. Even if you're doing everything 100% correct in terms of eating and avoiding toxins... it's almost impossible to escape the damage to your friendly gut bacteria. Our environment is too polluted. And so, you have to give them a helping hand.

The problem is, not all probiotics are created equal. Despite hundreds of products out there, few provide you with the full benefits of a true probiotic. And to understand why you have to know how these bacteria became so critical to our health in the first place.

For starters, all naturally occurring probiotics originate in the soil. And just like in your gut, they prevent the overgrowth of yeasts, molds, and other parasites. They also create a mineral rich environment and promote nutrient uptake. Without them, plants would rot and die.

Now, before pesticides and modern farming practices came along we had constant contact with these beneficial bacteria. For instance, we'd pull a carrot from the ground, wash it off a bit, and just eat it. And in doing so we'd invite these friendly microorganisms into our bodies. This helped keep us healthy by regulating our immune system. It also prevented yeast and other toxins from growing in our gut.

But these days, by the time your food ends up in the supermarket, it's been sterilized and lacks the good bugs. Additionally, pesticides destroy the soil's ecosystem, making the problem worse. Sadly, even many organic foods are devoid of these soil borne bacteria.

Because of this, our GI tract now lacks most of these naturally occurring bugs. We've lost that direct connection with nature and the bacteria that came with it. Consequently, our health is suffering. Sure, we might be living longer, but overall, we're sicker. And it makes perfect sense since 70% of our immune system is found in our gut and controlled by these microbes.

Now, the probiotics found in virtually every supplement are not the native bugs we evolved with throughout the years. Instead they're isolated strains that have been removed from their natural environment, individually cultured (often in a foreign medium), and then grouped back together into a packaged blend.

As a result, they come with key disadvantages...

For one, they're very sensitive to stomach acid. Therefore, most of them don't make it to your intestine where they're supposed to do their jobs. In fact, studies estimate that without specific protection, only 4% of the bacteria in your capsules survive. So, if you've ever bought a probiotic, there's a good chance that $0.96 out of every dollar you spent literally got flushed down the toilet.

Next, these bacterial strains are frozen dry before packaged into pill form. Because of this they're quite sensitive to heat and will die off without refrigeration. Unfortunately, that's what happens to products sitting on store shelves or while being delivered to you if you were to purchase them online.

In fact, an independent review by Consumer Labs indicated that some products contain as little as 16.3% of the amount of microorganisms claimed. So again, chances are you're wasting the majority of your money.

And what about the few that are refrigerated? Or shipped with ice packs? Well, consider the following: your body's temperature is 98.6 degrees Fahrenheit – far warmer than the temperature needed to keep these frozen bugs alive. So, what happens when they enter the hot environment of your body?

Something to think about...

Now, due to the drawbacks just discussed, supplement makers have come up with a metric known as CFU (or colony forming units). This is used to quantify the number of living organisms in a specific formulation. And since, in the mind of the consumer, "more equals better", companies try to one-up each other with higher and higher CFU's. You may have seen these on labels in the store: 5 billion CFU's, 10 billion CFU's, 15 billion CFU's...

But here's the rub...

What they don't tell you is that this number represents the number of live bacteria at the time of manufacture. By the time the product makes it to you, most of the bugs may already be dead. And that's before they even get to the harsh, acidic environment of your stomach.

Given these shortcomings, we decided to source our own probiotic that comes straight from the Earth and can withstand the harsh environment of the stomach to get to your intestines intact where it can do its job.

Furthermore, we added a couple of natural ingredients that support healthy blood sugar as new research has shown that the bad bugs in your gut cause blood sugar disturbances, which in turn lead to uncontrollable cravings and weight gain. The product is called SlimBiotine and you can learn more about it here:

GetSlimBiotine.com

XIII. Troubleshooting & Frequently Asked Questions

Almost everyone who starts this program experiences rapid and substantial weight loss within the first couple of weeks. In fact, I've had readers write in to report as much as 14 pounds in 14 days. Of course, this will vary from person to person.

In general, the more total weight you have to lose, the faster it will come off (at the beginning). And sure, most of this is water weight but it's still a good boost to your morale when you're getting on the scale and the numbers are quickly falling. It definitely motivates you to keep going.

With that said, there are exceptions to the above. Some people just don't respond initially, losing only one or two pounds during phase I. If this happens to you, **do not panic!** Stick with the program and the weight *will* start coming off during the second phase. Furthermore, you won't realize the full benefits of the CCD (and how much of a change it has made to your life) until a full 8 weeks have passed.

Now, be that as it may, let me explain the possible reasons you might not experience that initial weight loss most people do:

1. **You're eating too much**. This is a program that essentially forbids you from counting and portioning. As you know, the goal is to restore your natural hunger instinct to its working state so portion control becomes automatic.

   For some, this process doesn't happen immediately so they overeat in the first several days. That's fine and it will auto-correct itself after a couple of weeks (provided you're following the core program).

2. **Your insulin levels are too high**. This essentially ties in with the first reason. If your insulin levels are much higher than most people's, it will take a bit longer for them to drop and to get your natural hunger and appetite control mechanisms to be fully functional again. But don't let that deter you for a second.

   Stay on track, avoid sugars and carb-heavy meals, and it's going to happen, whether it takes one week, two weeks, or even three. Finally, if you haven't noticed any progress after three weeks (a very rare occurrence if you're following the program) send my team an Email to support@cruisecontroldiet.com so we can discuss this and figure out where the problem lies.

3. **You're not eating enough**. This is a big reason people fail to respond on The Cruise Control Diet. Look, just because it's called a diet doesn't mean you should be starving yourself. But that's exactly what many people do and it completely backfires.

Here's why...

Whenever you decrease your calories by eating less, your hormone levels begin to drop — specifically leptin and T4. And once their levels get low enough you stop losing weight.

It's a basic survival mechanism. Your body doesn't care that you want to slim down and look good. Its main purpose is keeping you alive. So, make sure you're giving your body what it needs.

Here's how to figure out if you're not eating enough (and what to do about it)...

First, click here to calculate your daily caloric needs on the CCD's website. Keep in mind, however, these are very rough estimates. That said, the calculators will give you a ballpark figure you should target.

Now, the best way to know if you're putting enough "fuel" into your body is to take note of your hunger and energy levels. In short, if you're feeling energetic throughout the day and you don't have cravings, you're on the right track.

On the other hand, if you get tired easily and you're "munchy"... you need to eat more quality food. And if this describes your scenario, here's how to fix it in a couple of days:

    i. Go off the program for 48 hours. Eat whatever your heart desires (heck, even binge). This will get your hormone levels back up to where you can start losing weight again.

    ii. After those 48 hours have passed, start over from Phase I again.

Now, a word of warning regarding the above: you may put on a few pounds during your binge. Not to worry, however. These will come off quite quick and the scale will continue trending downward. Just remember to eat enough quality food, and after Phase I is complete, enjoy your cheat meals 1-2 times per week.

4. **You have gut dysbiosis.** If you have trouble losing weight despite eating as the program prescribes, there's a good chance your intestines have been overrun with bad bacteria. At this point, taking a daily

probiotic (**getslimbiotine.com**), eating more fiber, and avoiding toxins as described in chapter XIII is highly recommended.

OK, with that out of the way, let's go over a few FAQ's I've gotten since I've released this program:

1. **Isn't this just another low-carb diet? How is it different from say, Atkins?**

   No, it's not another low-carb diet for a couple of reasons. For starters, it's a low-sugar, low-starch diet. You get tons of carbs on this program and you never go into ketosis.

   But there's a difference between the carbs you do get to eat. You have starchy carbs (e.g. potatoes) and fibrous carbs (e.g. cauliflower). And the latter are the staple of this program. You should eat them with every meal.

   Next, almost every other program requires you to count or keep track of something. This program doesn't. In fact, **it actually forbids you to do so.** Remember, you want to rely on instinct for weight maintenance not intellect. It's the only way to become a fit, healthy person as opposed to a (temporarily) thin dieter.

   Read that paragraph over several times until it sinks in. If you truly get it, you'll experience amazing results.

2. **Do I have to eat a lot of meat?**

   Absolutely not. Vegetables should be a big part of daily caloric intake. Personally I love meat so I eat it in larger quantities. I've also taken up powerlifting as of late so I need the protein. Your activity levels (and hence, nutritional needs) are probably different. And if that's the case you can lower your portions accordingly.

3. **I'm a bit constipated since I started this diet, what should I do?**

   Changing your diet (especially if the change is a far cry from what you're used to) will naturally alter your bowel movements. But not to worry, this is only temporary. As long as you're eating enough vegetables and staying hydrated everything will go back to normal within a few weeks.

In the meantime, however, feel free to help things along somewhat. The best way to do this is by eating prunes. I've never come across a more powerful (natural) laxative. I'm sure they exist, but this has always worked wonders for me.

A final note regarding prunes... I know I've essentially made dried fruits off limits. This is the only exception. Use them sparingly to help you get over this hump. Then, lay off them altogether and stick to their fresh counterparts (i.e. plums).

And that does it for this section. Be sure to get in touch if you have questions I haven't covered.

XIV. Conclusion

While we've come to the end of the book, in reality, this is just the beginning. My hope is that you take the concepts outlined in these pages and use them as a springboard to continue bettering your health.

I'll shoot you updates from time to time regarding topics that concern fitness and nutrition. You might get an Email once a week or once a month. It all depends on what I come across on any given day and if it's worth sharing.

So, in closing, I wish you the best of success with your weight loss efforts and health overall. This won't be a walk in the park but as you'll see, it's not that hard either.

Stick with it and it won't be long before you're looking back to this very moment... full of pride for having seen this through till the end... and in the best shape you've been in years (perhaps ever).

Now, get to it!

To Your Health,

James Ward

XV. Recommended Resources

1. ## SlimBiotine

   Few supplements have as big of an impact on your weight (*and health overall*) as a quality probiotic. But they're not all created equal. You need one that can withstand the harsh, acidic environment of your stomach and reach your intestines to do its job.

2. ## Why We Get Fat: And What To Do About It

   This is arguably (along with the pedometer) one of the most important resources in this list. In fact, it's not just recommended – **it's required reading**!

   If I had to pick one thing to attribute my dramatic transformation from fat to fit to (along with supreme health) then this book is definitely it.

   Written by Gary Taubes, it challenges the conventional calories-in/calories-out paradigm and presents an alternative hypothesis backed by multiple medical studies as well as anecdotal evidence. It's a truly eye-opening read and should be in everyone's library.

3. ## Food Inc.

   A chilling, yet eye-opening documentary about the sad state of the food industry. Like mentioned earlier in this book, nothing will motivate you to start shopping local and organic more than seeing how things really are behind the scenes. Please take the time to watch this.

4. ## Fat Head

   This is a very entertaining yet highly informative (and well researched) documentary put together by comedian Tom Naughton. It's his "response" to the popular documentary, *Super Size Me*.

   In a nutshell, Naughton successfully dispels the common notion that fast food is to blame for our bulging waistlines. In fact, he went on to lose several pounds while eating nothing but McDonald's for a month. Furthermore, all of his health indicators improved.

   Naughton also touches upon a lot of the material covered in this book.

The Cruise Control Diet
COOK BOOK

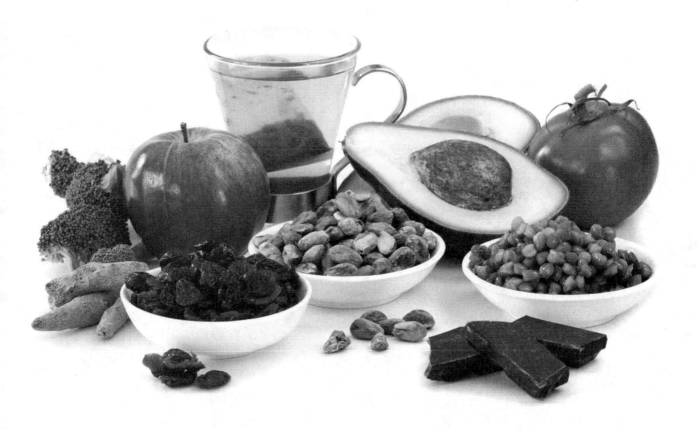

JAMES WARD

Table of Contents

I. Introduction

This book contains a collection of meals that I eat on a regular basis. They were compiled from a number of different sources including cookbooks, the Internet, friends and family... and a bit of experimentation ☺

Now, if you don't usually cook, the task may seem a bit daunting. But don't sweat it. All of these are meant for a beginner in the kitchen. And as you'll soon discover, they'll form a springboard of ideas for your very own recipes down the road.

Learning to prepare easy meals at home is the key to following a healthy diet. If you don't have a good cooked meal and no idea how to quickly put one together, you'll inevitably slip and order that pizza (or hit the local burger joint).

You should know that most take-out foods are made with poor quality meats and veggies. They typically come from questionable sources. They're also packed with sugars, starches, and who knows what else. This is not an option any more... at least not on a daily basis (cheat meals are a different story).

Furthermore, most of the low-carb (or better stated, low-starch) recipes you'll find online aren't very satisfying. They're essentially stripped down versions of traditional meals. But since they lack the usual fattening garnishes and other ingredients, they end up quite tasteless.

On the contrary, the following recipes are in their original forms (i.e. they were never meant to be cooked with starches and sugars in the first place). So, **you don't end up sacrificing taste for health**. And that's crucial, because becoming bored with your everyday food is the kiss of death when it comes to dieting.

One last thing regarding these recipes: some of them are a bit adventurous (e.g. lamb steaks). Obviously, if this is beyond your taste preferences, you don't have to eat them. None of these foods here are essential provided you're following the low-starch, low-sugar rules. Again, they're just food for thought (pun intended).

Alright, now before we dig in, let's take a moment to go over some basic kitchen equipment you'll need. You don't need a lot but there are some essentials...

- Paella pan (with lid) – This is essentially a deep and wide pan that is used for making omelets, bacon, to stir fry veggies, sauté onions, as well as to slow cook meat in a little liquid (braising).

- Casserole – ceramic, with or without a lid. Good for baking meals, reheating food in the oven, and also for serving.

- Wide boiling pot – a pot that is also oven safe is very useful. You can use it for soups, for slow cooking in the oven, and for making pot roast. A wider one will be more useful because it can accommodate larger meats when they need to be cooking without overlapping.

- Meat tongs – these are essential for handling hot meat. You simply can't do it without these.

- Salad spinner – your salads will taste ten times better if the veggies are not wet and soggy (but rather crisp and dry)... especially when making leafy salads like spinach and lettuce. Sure, you can wash and pat dry each leaf individually but it takes forever. A salad spinner will help you put everything together in no time.

- Hand held blender – there are many varieties of soup blenders but there is no need to buy expensive machines. One small handheld blender is enough. You will be blending only boiled and roasted veggies to make a sauce or a dip. No need for heavy-duty blenders.

- Meat thermometer – you can find a decent electronic instant meat thermometer for $10-15. It will help you determine whether your meat is ready, especially if you don't have much experience or when making a recipe for the first time.

- Big wooden cutting board and cutting knife – you'll be chopping veggies daily. Get yourself a decent board that will make this easy for you.

- A cooking apron!

Alright, on to the actual recipes...

II. Recipes

A. Salads

The secret to a good salad is not so much the particular ingredients or that "special" dressing, but the fresh vegetables. An organic, locally grown, recently picked tomato on the vine has a completely different taste than a conventionally grown greenhouse tomato (night and day difference!).

Unfortunately, these vegetables aren't very cheap. A good organic cucumber can go for up to $2. The same goes for the high quality local peppers.

But it's understandable. These perishables are harvested fresh with no preservatives and are meant to reach your table within a few days. So, resist the urge to be stingy with your veggies on this.

In fact, you'll probably end up spending the same amount of money on vegetables as you do on meat. And while the meat is much more caloric (i.e. more "value" for your dollar) keep in mind that the vegetables provide the minerals and micronutrients that allow for those calories to be utilized to the max.

You'll see that when you start eating a good-sized salad with every meal, you'll experience a burst of energy like never before (much different from the typical crash of a starch-heavy meal). Fresh and raw is the name of the game here.

Now, a word about salad dressings...

Many of us of are "trained" when making a salad to reach for a bottle with the label "salad dressing" to pour over. First of all, most of these are packed with the exact things we are trying to avoid (i.e. sugar and preservatives).

Secondly, you will discover that most salads are perfectly delicious with nothing more than a little olive oil, lemon, and/or vinegar. Salt, black pepper, and oregano are also commonly added to salads to make them even tastier.

You should already have these ingredients in your kitchen. There is absolutely no need to buy any type of salad dressing (unless you have a specific recipe you like and follow).

And trust me... **you will not miss ranch, or creamy, or whatever else you are used to.** If the salad requires a cheesy taste, just add good old original feta or any other creamy cheese that you like.

The ingredient quantities are for a good-sized personal salad. Double everything if you have a meal companion (or triple, quadruple if feeding a family).

Greek Village Salad

Ingredients:

1 tomato on the vine
1 cucumber (or half if using the long ones)
½ green bell pepper (also good with 1 green Italian pepper)
½ of a small onion
Feta cheese
Olives
Salt
Black pepper
Oregano
Parsley (optional)
Olive oil

Cut the tomato and pepper into big bites, the cucumber into semi-circles, and slice the onion into long, thin strips. Add olives as you like and put a thin rectangle of feta on top.

Sprinkle with olive oil (2-3 tbsps.), salt, black pepper, oregano, and chopped parsley (if using). Some people like it with ½ teaspoon of vinegar. I eat it without. As with every recipe, experiment to your liking.

This is absolutely delicious and you will find yourself craving this refreshing salad every day. For additional flavor, add some capers as well.

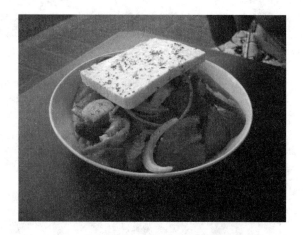

Lettuce Salads

Lettuce salads are traditionally made with green leaf or Romaine lettuce. It is a good practice to mix in some other greens such as baby spring mix, red leaf, mesclun, oak leaf lettuce, Boston lettuce, arugula, radicchio, endive, etc... the list is endless.

The only lettuce you should not use is the iceberg, simply because it has such a poor nutrient content compared to any of the above. You'll also find that after eating the aforementioned greens, iceberg will seem completely tasteless and undesirable to you.

Finally, a good practice is to add a few leaves of spinach to your lettuce. Many people have a hard time consuming raw spinach. But when it's mixed this way on regular basis... it gives you 100% of its nutritional value in raw form without having to make a spinach salad by itself.

Basic Lettuce Salad

Ingredients:

½ head of romaine lettuce
1 cucumber (1/2 if using long cucumbers)
½ green bell pepper (or 1 full Italian pepper)

Wash the lettuce leaves individually and spin them to dry well, or pat dry. Chop lettuce, cucumber and green pepper. Mix together, add olive oil (about 2 tbsp.) and vinegar (about 1 tbsp.), salt, black pepper, oregano.

Rich Lettuce Salad

In addition to the above, you can make your salad richer by adding:

- A few leaves of a different type of lettuce
- Scallions
- Plenty of dill (some love it just basic with a ton of dill)
- Red radish (finely chopped)
- A few leaves of spinach
- Red or yellow pepper instead of green
- Cherry tomatoes
- Olives

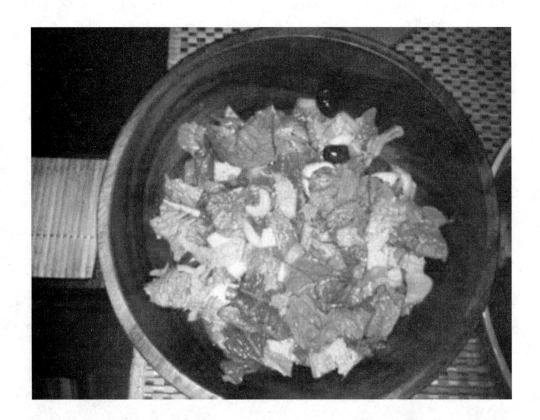

Peppers and Portabella Salad

Ingredients:

½ red bell pepper
½ green bell pepper
½ orange or yellow bell pepper
1 fresh portabella mushroom cap
3-4 leaves of romaine lettuce
Feta cheese
Salt
Black pepper
½ of a small onion (optional)

Cut the peppers into long slices. Cut the mushroom cap into long thin slices as well. Chop the lettuce. Slice the onion into long thin strings (if using). Add salt, black pepper, 1 tbsp. of vinegar, and 1 tbsp. of olive oil. Crumble the feta on top. This salad is very filling and colorful!

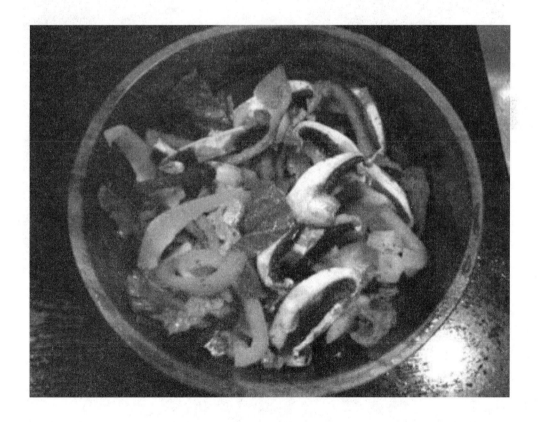

Spinach Salad With Walnuts and Goat Cheese

Ingredients:

Fresh baby spinach (enough to fill your salad bowl)
Roughly chopped walnuts
Goat cheese
Balsamic vinegar
Grape tomatoes (optional)

Wash the spinach leaves well and spin or pat dry. The goat cheese can be replaced with feta if needed (or any other white creamy cheese for that matter). Any tomato goes well with this. Sprinkle with very little (i.e. 1 tsp.) of balsamic vinegar and mix well.

WARNING: Be very careful with the balsamic. A little too much and you will spoil the whole salad!

Basic Tomato Salad

Ingredients:

1-2 tomatoes on the vine
Salt
Black pepper
Oregano
Basil (optional)
Parsley (optional)
Feta cheese (optional)

This is more of a vegetable side dish than a real salad. All you need to do is cut the tomatoes any way you please, sprinkle olive oil, salt, black pepper, and plenty of oregano. You can also add chopped parsley, basil, or feta if you so desire.

Cabbage Carrot Salad

Ingredients:

1/3 of a green cabbage head (small size)
3 carrots
Dill
Lemon

Shred the cabbage. Grate the carrots over it. Chop some dill and squeeze half of a lemon (or more) on top. Season with salt. Nothing else needed!

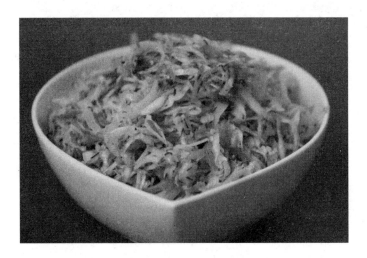

Cabbage Dill Salad

This salad might seem very similar to the previous, yet the taste is very different.

Ingredients:

1/3 of a green cabbage head (small size)
Dill

Chop the cabbage into long strings. Add about a tbsp. of salt and mash well with your hands for a few minutes. Add chopped dill and season with olive oil and vinegar.

Roast Pepper Salad

Ingredients:

3 peppers of your favorite kind (e.g. bell peppers, Italian peppers; any color)
1 spoon crumbled feta
1 spoon chopped parsley
1 garlic clove (optional)

Place the peppers in a baking dish. Turn the oven to broil and roast the peppers turning them from time to time until black on all sides.

Place in a bag or a container with a lid and close. Let them "suffocate" and cool. When cool enough to handle, peel the skin, remove the stem and seeds, and chop the "meat" into bite-sized pieces. Season with lots of salt, 2 tablespoons of olive oil, and about 1 tablespoon of red wine vinegar. Sprinkle with parsley, feta, and finely chopped garlic (if using).

Beats With Arugula (or Baby Spring Mix)

If you make this salad for your family, I guarantee you it will make you look like a gourmet chef! This is the type of food high-end restaurants charge hefty prices for and serve small portions of. It is very healthy for you, has rich colors, and the taste is addictive.

Ingredients:

2 small to medium red beets
1-2 oz. arugula (or baby spring mix if arugula is not to your taste)
Goat cheese to garnish
Walnuts to taste

For the dressing:

¼ cup olive oil
Juice from ½ lemon
¼ teaspoon powdered mustard

Boil the red beets vigorously for about 30-45 min. They need to be soft enough for a fork to go through them. Let them cool and chop them into slices, cubes, or any other shape you like (e.g. long strings). This step can be done ahead of time and the beets placed in the fridge.

Prepare the dressing separately by adding all dressing ingredients together. Then add the walnuts, red beets, and dressing to the arugula. Mix very well. Ideally, you want to put everything in a closed container and shake well.

Serve garnished with the goat cheese. Add the salt and pepper directly at the end to your taste.

Tuna Salad

This is a great lunch when there is nothing prepared and no time to cook. It is a good idea to keep tuna cans for days like this.

Ingredients:

1 can of tuna
1 tbsp. of mayonnaise
½ lemon
1 tomato
1 celery stick
Lettuce

Open the tuna can, squeeze as much water out of the can as possible, and empty into a mixing bowl.

Chop the tomato and celery and add them to the tuna. Put in the mayonnaise, squeeze the lemon on top, and season well with salt and black pepper to taste. Mix well.

Place the tuna mix over a bed of chopped lettuce.

Lettuce Avocado Salad

Ingredients:

½ head of lettuce
2 avocados (ripe: soft at the very ends, hard at the center)
1 small cucumber
1 tsp. balsamic vinegar
Crumbled feta (optional)

Chop the lettuce. Cut the avocadoes in half resulting in two long halves – one of which contains the pit. Remove the pit with a spoon. Use the spoon to scoop out the avocado from the skin. Slice the avocado in long cuts and add to the lettuce. Cut the cucumber in circles and add it as well. Add the feta if using. Season with salt, pepper, 2 tablespoons of olive oil, and about 1 teaspoon of balsamic vinegar. Mix well.

Lettuce Avocado Salad With Pear and Walnuts

Ingredients:

½ lettuce head
1 small cucumber
1 avocado (ripe: soft at the very ends, hard at the center)
1 pear (make sure it is hard and crispy, not soft)
1 tbsp. walnuts
1 tbsp. crumbled feta or blue cheese
1 tsp. balsamic vinegar

Chop the lettuce and cucumber. Cut the avocado in half, remove the pit with a spoon, scoop out the two halves and chop them into the salad. Cut the pear in slices and add that too. Season with salt, 1 tsp. balsamic vinegar, and 1 tbsp. olive oil. Spread the walnuts and cheese on top.

Alfalfa Spouts Salad

You might not know what Alfalfa spouts are but if your local store happens to have them, they will become a weekly favorite. You'll find them where the fresh lettuce is in your supermarket. They usually come in a 4 oz. container pre-washed and ready to go. This salad is very crunchy and refreshing. It is useful for a midweek salad when you are too busy to prepare anything complicated.

Ingredients:

4 oz. Alfalfa sprouts package
½ cucumber
4-5 cherry tomatoes

Combine the spouts with the chopped cucumber, cherry tomatoes, and nothing else. Spice with a tablespoon of olive oil and a teaspoon of balsamic vinegar. Add salt if needed.

B. Vegetable Side Dishes

Making the same salad every day as a side dish will work for some time, but eventually, you'll get bored and want something different. A good variety of vegetables, uncooked or minimally cooked, are essential and you'll find yourself always looking for a new vegetable to make as a side dish.

These are my top 13...

Roasted Brussels Sprouts

Wash the sprouts well. Cut the ends slightly if you'd like (this is not really necessary; it's simply to remove the brown part). You can also cut the big ones in half – or even quarters. Place them in a big mixing bowl and coat slightly with olive oil. Sprinkle salt on top and mix them well with a spoon.

Preheat the oven at 400F. Place the sprouts on a baking sheet making sure they are evenly laid out and not on top of each other. Put them in the oven for about 10 minutes. At this point, you will see them start to brown. You can shake the pan a little and let them roast longer if you prefer them crispier.

Roasted Brussels sprouts are delicious served immediately hot, or even cold the following day.

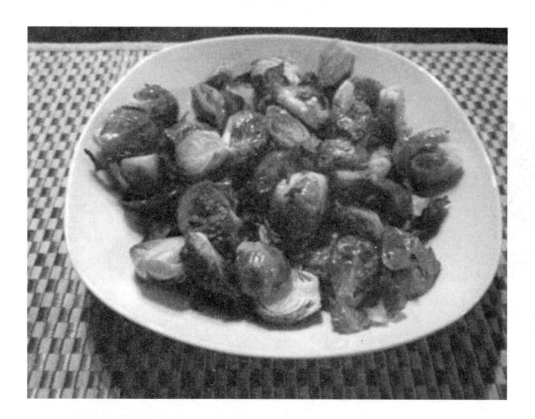

Broccoli

Cut the heads into bite-sized pieces and toss well with lemon and olive oil. No other spices are needed. I prefer to eat my broccoli raw. However, if you find that is too crunchy for your liking, you can boil it for 5-10 minutes before adding the olive oil and lemon.

Also, don't throw away the stalks! They can be just as delicious as the florets. All you need to do is boil them in water for a few minutes until they are soft when pierced with a fork (these are not so good raw... far too "fibrous"). Then, slice them in circles and mix well with freshly squeezed lemon and olive oil.

Cauliflower

You can prepare cauliflower exactly the same way as broccoli.

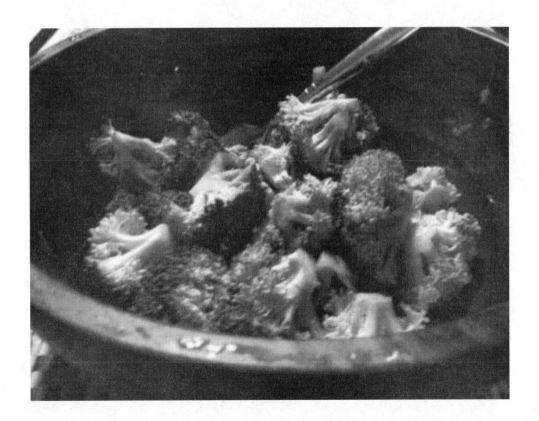

Green Beans

Ingredients:

½ lb. green beans
3 garlic cloves

Slightly trim the thick end of the beans. Next, wash and towel dry them. Chop the garlic into fine pieces. Then, mix the beans and the garlic in a bowl and sprinkle with some salt and olive oil. Toss them well so that all beans are evenly coated with the oil, salt, and garlic.

Preheat the oven at 400F. Place the beans on a baking sheet in a single layer. Roast for 5-6 minutes. If you like them very crispy, at this point switch the oven to broil and brown them a little. These are good served immediately but can also be eaten chilled at a later time.

You could also prepare these on the stovetop. Just preheat some olive oil on medium heat and cook the beans that way. You might want to cover the pan because there will be a lot of spatter.

Roasted Peppers and Onions

Ingredients:

1 medium onion
2 bell peppers (any color)

Roughly chop the bell peppers. Chop the onion in skewer-sized pieces. Mix everything together and brown with olive oil, salt, lots of black pepper, and oregano.

Next, put them in the oven to broil for about 10 minutes, stirring and tossing them as needed to achieve a crisp browning on all sides. Serve immediately.

Spinach

This is a simple, yet delicious, spinach recipe. I can't get enough of this one (and you won't either). Actually, you'll be surprised how easily you can literally *devour* large quantities of this super food when slightly cooked like this.

Ingredients:

1/2 lb. fresh spinach
4 garlic cloves (chopped, finely)
1 tbsp. butter
2 tbsp. feta cheese (optional)

Wash and drain the spinach well. Don't cut its stems off and don't chop it either. Heat butter in a frying pan on medium low heat. Add the chopped garlic and sauté for 1 minute. Add the spinach and mix well.

Cover and let everything sauté on low heat for 1-2 minutes. If you're planning on having this with feta, add it now and mix well. Sauté for another minute. Serve immediately hot.

If you're not using feta, add salt to taste. Otherwise, the feta will confer enough saltiness to the spinach to forgo the salt.

Bok Choy Stir Fry

Bok Choy (also known as leafy Chinese cabbage) is one of the most common vegetables in Asia. It's a great addition to your repertoire of recipes for variety.

Ingredients:

1 Bok Choy
2 scallions
3 garlic cloves (chopped)
1 small onion (chopped)
A handful of peanuts
Pure sesame oil

Heat olive oil on medium heat and sauté the onion and garlic for about 4 minutes. Add roughly chopped Bok Choy and scallions, sprinkle with sesame oil, and mix well. Continue to sauté for another 2 minutes until the vegetable slightly softens. Serve immediately with peanuts sprinkled on top (walnuts work great as well).

Red Pepper

This is more of an idea than an actual recipe. Red peppers can be a side meal or served on their own. This holds especially true when you're packing a lunch on the go. As you know, it's fine to use previously cooked meat and just reheat it. However, previously cooked vegetables are never as tasty.

You'll find that big bell peppers are very filling on their own. Just wash and cut into long strips. You can add a block of feta with them, or any one of your favorite cheeses for that matter.

If you've been off the sugar long enough, you'll find that your taste buds have become increasingly sensitive to sweet flavors. Thus, the pepper will taste pleasantly sweet – no salt or other spices are needed!

Roasted Eggplant

These are best prepared on a BBQ grill. They really taste different when made on the grill vs. the oven. However, even if you don't have access to a grill, they'll still come out quite delicious.

Use baby eggplants for best taste. Slice them into circles or ovals (about as thick as you would a slice of bread). Coat with olive oil. Put on the grill or on a baking sheet at 400F. For faster results, make sure your oven is already preheated. When browned, flip over.

Season with salt and serve immediately (or cold later). You can garnish with chopped parsley, feta cheese, and/or garlic.

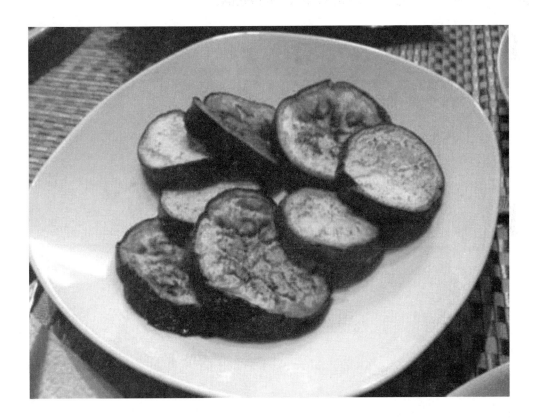

Asparagus

Chop any rough, thick ends and discard. In a mixing bowl, coat well with olive oil and salt. You can also add some minced garlic.

Now, these can be made in three different ways:

1. On the grill for about 5 minutes.

2. In the oven at 400F on a baking sheet for 5-10 minutes.

3. In a sauté pan with butter or olive oil, covered, at medium high heat. Stir them regularly until they start to brown. Make sure not to overcook them or they will get sour.

Eggplant Dip

There are as many variations of this spread as there are of bruschetta spreads in Italy. Eggplant dips are popular all over the Mediterranean countries. It is a great side to a meal or as an appetizer. It can be stored in the refrigerator for up to 10 days and is always served cold.

Ingredients:

2 green tomatoes
1 red pepper
1 eggplants, medium size
3 garlic cloves
½ cup parsley
½ boiled carrot (optional)

Boil the carrot (if you plan on using it). Preheat the oven at 400F and roast the pepper and eggplant. You can even roast the garlic for a little just to soften it.

Once the veggies are well browned on all sides, wrap them in a paper towel and let them "suffocate" and cool down. As soon as they're ready to handle, peel the pepper and chop it. Chop the garlic as well. Scoop the inside of the eggplant with a spoon.

Mix everything together: the scooped eggplant, the roasted chopped pepper, chopped garlic, green tomatoes, parsley, and carrot.

Puree everything together with a blender. Add a drop of olive oil and a drop of red wine vinegar. Serve garnished with fresh parsley.

You can also add a little bit of the eggplant peel to the mix. This gives the spread a unique smoky taste. This is especially tasty if the eggplants were roasted on the grill.

Guacamole

Ingredients:

2 ripe avocados (ends only should be soft to touch, the rest should still be firm)
1/2 tomato
1/2 lime
Cilantro (optional)

Cut the avocados in half and scoop out with a spoon. Chop the tomato finely (and the cilantro, if using) and add to the avocado. Squeeze the lime on top. Season very well with salt. Mix well. You want to end up with a chunky guacamole, not creamy, so don't use a blender, just a fork to mush everything together.

This is best if eaten immediately. It is very filling and makes an excellent side dish or snack on it's own.

Roasted Mushrooms

Ingredients:

¾ lb. crimini mushrooms
1 spring of fresh rosemary or ½ tsp. dry
2-3 springs fresh thyme or 1 tsp. dry
Juice from 1/3 lemon
1 tbsp. olive oil

Preheat the oven at 350F. Mix everything in a bowl. Add salt and pepper to taste. Place on a baking dish and leave in the oven for 30 minutes. Serve immediately.

Cook Book

Zucchini and Summer Squash

This is an absolutely delicious and simple side dish that is best prepared on the grill. Here is how to do it using the oven.

Turn the broil on to high. Slice the veggies in ¼ inch circles. Season with olive oil and salt, mix well, and layer on a baking dish. Place them in the broiler for 3-4 minutes (or until they start to brown), turn them over, and leave them in for another 2-3 minutes.

Eggplant Parmesan

This recipe calls for a lot of cheese. Dairy is a gray area in terms of weight loss. Some people can eat a lot of it and still continue to lose weight while others find that not to be the case.

Either way, this fulfilling recipe is great for the summer months when you have fresh eggplants from the market. It goes really well with a green salad.

Prep time: 20 min.   Cook time: 20 min.

Ingredients:

2 large eggplants
24 oz. tomato sauce
2 cups grated Mozzarella cheese
½ cup grated Parmesan cheese

Preheat the oven at 400F.

Cut the eggplants in slices, about ½ inch thick. You need to pre-cook the slices either on the grill or in the oven for about 15 minutes on each side. Make sure you brush the eggplants with olive oil so they don't stick and burn.

Grease a baking dish with olive oil and place the following layers: eggplant, tomato sauce, cheese. Repeat 2-3 times. Cook for about 20 minutes, uncovered, until the cheese on top starts to brown.

C. Soups

There are countless delicious soup recipes out there and I encourage you to find new ones and experiment. I've included a few here that are great to eat in the fall and winter. But, treat them as appetizers as they'll probably not keep you full.

A side note on vegetable soups: it's best to eat your vegetables raw or minimally cooked. When heated (even slightly) they lose some of their nutritional value. Therefore, it is best if you do not try to get your servings of veggies from soups.

Fresh Tomato Soup

This is a delicious summer soup and should only be made with fresh ripe tomatoes.

Ingredients:

2 red peppers
2 carrots
1 lb. fresh tomatoes
1 small onion
2 garlic cloves
½ cup fresh basil

Roast the red peppers on a baking sheet at 400F. Turn as needed so they brown well. When well roasted, wrap them in a towel to "suffocate" and set aside (this makes peeling the skin easier when they cool off).

Chop the onion, garlic, carrot, and basil and sauté in olive oil until translucent. Start sautéing the onion and carrot; add the garlic in a few minutes later. 2 minutes later, add the basil.

In the meantime, bring water to a boil and drop the tomatoes in for 1 minute. You will see the skin of the tomato start to break apart. At this point, take them out of the water with a slotted spoon. Let them cool and peel the skin off.

Add the peeled, chopped tomatoes and red peppers to the sautéed veggies. Add a cup of water, bring to a boil, and simmer for 30 minutes. Allow to cool slightly and blend everything with a soup blender. Season with salt and black pepper.

Serve hot or cold with fresh basil on top.

Russian Spring Soup

This soup is a rich "vegetable bomb" – a meal in itself. Don't be discouraged by the large number of different ingredients. You should already have most of these in your home since they are commonly used in salads and other recipes. The most time consuming part is washing and chopping all of the veggies.

Prep time: 20 min.   Cook time: 30 min.

Ingredients:

1 onion
1 garlic glove
1 small turnip
1 small parsnip
2 carrots
1 celery stick
4 cups stock (chicken or vegetable)
7 oz. fresh spinach (about a bowl)
Fresh dill
Parsley
1 lemon
1 egg

This soup is very straightforward. All you have to do is boil everything together, add the more delicate spinach and dill at the end, and finally garnish.

Here we go...

Cut the onion, turnip, parsnip, carrots, and celery into bite-sized chunks. Chop the garlic glove. Add everything in the stock and bring to a boil. Then, simmer for 25 minutes.

Next, add the roughly chopped spinach and simmer for another 5 minutes. You want to keep this power vegetable fresh and green. This is why we only add it at the end.

Season well with salt and black pepper to taste. Serve while hot and garnish with dill and parsley. Squeeze fresh lemon juice right in the bowl. Place 1 boiled egg cut in quarters.

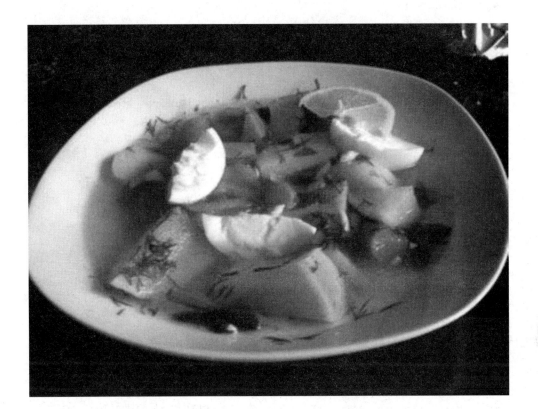

Chicken Soup

Here is my version of a delicious chicken soup that you can make in no time.

Prep time: 10 min.   Cook time: 30 min.

Ingredients:

4 chicken thighs (this is by far the tastiest cut choice for a soup)
2 carrots
1 celery stick
1 large onion
750 ml. chicken stock
1 lemon
Parsley
2 eggs

Chop the onion and carrots and sauté in olive oil until translucent. Add the chicken pieces and stir for about 1 minute. Add the chopped celery and pour in the chicken stock. Bring to boil. Lower the temperature, add salt and black pepper to taste, and simmer for about 30 minutes.

When the meat is ready, fish it out, let it cool, cut into bite-sized pieces and remove the bones (if you used bone-in thighs).

In the meantime, cream the rest. A soup blender works best here if you have one. This makes the soup thicker without the traditional use of rice or flour. Bring the meat pieces back inside. Alternatively, if you want to have some veggies visible in the soup, you can separate and cream only half of the soup. This will leave some of the carrot and celery pieces visible for color.

Adding the eggs: take a cup of the cooked soup base and set aside to cool. Beat two eggs with a fork in a bowl. Wait until the liquid is cool enough so not to clump the eggs (you can test this by adding a drop of your well beaten eggs into the liquid and see if it clumps up).

Add the beaten eggs slowly into the cooled liquid while stirring. Add the mixture to the soup. Serve immediately. Squeeze half a lemon or less into each bowl and garnish with fresh parsley and black pepper.

Meat Balls Soup

This soup is originally from Cyprus and is a fantastic source of protein. The original recipe is with lamb, but can be made with any cut. If you don't like or eat pork, try it with ground beef or ground turkey.

Prep time: 10 min.   Cook time: 60 min.

Ingredients:

1 lb. ground pork
1 medium/small onion
¼ cup fresh parsley
3 eggs
32 oz. chicken stock
1 lemon

In a large bowl, mix the ground meat, one of the eggs, and the parsley well with your hands. Season with salt and black pepper and continue mixing. Shape into walnut size balls and set aside.

Bring the chicken stock to a boil, drop the balls in, and reduce to a simmer. After an hour, take a ladle of the liquid (about 1 cup) and set aside to cool.

Beat the remaining two eggs very well. When the liquid has cooled down, slowly add the eggs while mixing well. You don't want the heat of the liquid to clump up the eggs. Add the juice of one lemon.

Now, add this all back to the soup. Let it sit covered for a couple of minutes (or on low simmer) to allow the eggs to cook.

Serve hot with some fresh parsley and black pepper on top. Add more squeezed lemon juice if desired.

Mushroom Soup

This soup has a very soothing flavor. Mix 2-3 types of mushrooms for best results e.g. cremini, shiitake, Oyster mushrooms, etc.

Prep time: 10 min.   Cook time: 20 min.

Ingredients:

20 oz. fresh mushrooms (to make about 8 cups when sliced)
1 medium onion
4 tbsp. butter
½ cup dry white wine
3 cups heavy cream
64 oz. chicken stock
2 bay leaves
Fresh chives to garnish, optional

Spices:

¼ tsp. nutmeg
½ tsp. dried thyme (or 1 tsp. fresh)
1 tsp. salt
1 tsp. black pepper

In a saucepan, melt the butter, and add the bay leaves. Chop the onion and sauté in the butter until translucent.

Add the mushrooms, stir well, and cook for another 5 minutes or until they soften. Add all spices and mix well.

Pour in the chicken stock and stir again. Pour in the cream, mix well, and bring to boil. Reduce heat immediately and let it simmer at low temperature for another 10 minutes.

Serve hot with freshly chopped chives on top and some more black pepper. Add additional salt as needed.

Cream of Mushroom Soup

If you like soups, here is another way to prepare a mushroom soup with almost the same ingredients as above. Again, for best flavor, mix different types of fresh mushrooms. This time you roast the mushrooms first.

Prep time: 45 min.   Cook time: 10 min.

Ingredients:

1 lb. fresh mushrooms
1 medium onion
32 oz. vegetable stock
8 oz. heavy cream
2 garlic cloves
Fresh thyme

Spices:

1 tsp. dried thyme (or 2 tsp. fresh)
½ tsp. dried sage (or 1 tsp. fresh)

Preheat oven at 400F.

Chop the mushrooms and place them in a large mixing bowl. Toss well with 1-2 tablespoons of olive oil and spice well with half the thyme, salt, and pepper to taste. Mix well. Place on a baking sheet and bake in the oven for 30-40 minutes or until they start to brown.

In a heavy pan, heat 2 tablespoons of olive oil, chop the onion, and sauté until translucent for about 5 minutes. Chop the garlic and add it to the onion together with the remaining thyme and the sage. Turn off the heat and wait for the mushrooms to be done.

Once roasted, add the mushrooms to the pan and pour in the vegetable broth. Bring to a boil and then reduce immediately. Let it simmer for 10 minutes at low heat.

Remove from the heat and blend with a hand blender. Serve immediately and garnish with fresh thyme.

Cream of Broccoli Soup

Once you make a few of these cream soups you will realize you can blend and make a cream soup from almost any vegetable. Here is how to make a cream soup out of broccoli. Notice the similarities with the mushrooms soups.

Prep time: 5 min.   Cook time: 60 min.

Ingredients:

8 cups of chopped broccoli florets (about 4 lbs.)
1 medium onion
3 tablespoons butter
4 celery sticks
12 oz. chicken stock
16 oz. heavy whipping cream
2 teaspoons garlic salt

Start by chopping the onion and celery. In a heavy pot, melt the butter and add the chopped onion and celery. Sautee for about 5-7 minutes until the onion is translucent. Add all other ingredients to the pot – all broccoli, broth, garlic, salt and black pepper. Bring to a boil, reduce the heat, and simmer for about 45 minutes. Stir in the cream and cook for another 10 minutes. Serve immediately.

Cream of Onion Soup

Prep time: 70 min.   Cook time: 20 min.

Ingredients:

1.5 lb. Vidalia onions
1 whole garlic head
28 oz. vegetable stock
1 bay leaf
1/8 teaspoon saffron, if using
3 teaspoons dry sherry or any type of sweet wine
¼ teaspoon black pepper
1/8 teaspoon salt
Shredded Swiss cheese to garnish

Preheat oven at 375F.

Cut the onions into quarters. Break the garlic head into individual cloves but don't peel them. Put them in small pouch of aluminum foil, drizzle olive oil to crease them slightly, and wrap fully in the aluminum foil.

Grease a baking sheet with olive oil. Spread the onion cuts on top and place the aluminum wrapped garlic on the baking sheet as well. Bake for 30 minutes, turn the onions over and then bake for another 30 minutes.

When ready, let them cool for about 10 minutes. In a heavy pan, squeeze the garlic out of the skin, and then add the onion and all other ingredients. Bring to a boil and then immediately reduce the heat to medium low. Simmer for 15 minutes.

Let it cool a little and then blend with a hand blender. Start the heat again to warm the soup up, add an additional tablespoon of sherry, and squeeze ½ lemon in.

Serve immediately with shredded Swiss cheese to garnish.

Plain Cabbage Soup

Don't be misled by the simplicity of this recipe. It is a perfect meal for an afternoon winter snack or as a warm appetizer to a meal. It is a favorite with children and even people who do not like cabbage will beg you to make it again.

Prep time: 5 min.   Cook time: 60 min.

Ingredients:

¼ cup butter
1 large white cabbage, shredded
1 ½ quarts chicken stock
1 tsp. salt
½ tsp. pepper
1/8 tsp. allspice

You will need a large pot as shredded cabbage takes a lot of volume. Start by melting the butter. Add the cabbage and cook for 3 minutes, stirring constantly to coat well with the butter. Add the remaining ingredients. Simmer covered for about 1 hour.

Serve warm.

D. Meats

If you have a barbeque, this will be the easiest section of your meal preparation. All you need to do is throw something on the grill and cut yourself a salad (or make one of the vegetable side dishes). If you don't have a grill or would like something different, the recipes below are easy to follow.

It is important to mention again here that pretty much every pre-packaged marinade out there is also pre-loaded with sugar. Do not be tempted to add any barbeque sauce or other condiments. Marinade your meats only with ingredients you put together yourself.

Braised Spareribs

OK, we all know spare ribs are delicious when marinated in barbeque and other sauces. So, how can we preserve that mouth-watering taste while avoiding sugar? The answer is to load this meal with different spices and cook it slowly. Here we go:

Prep time: 30 min.   Cook time: 2 hrs.

Ingredients:

2.5 lbs. spareribs
1 medium onion
2 cloves of garlic
14 oz. chopped tomatoes can (or 2 fresh medium tomatoes, chopped)
½ cup red wine
¼ cup parsley
1 bay leaf
1/8 tsp. cinnamon
1/8 tsp. ground cloves
1/8 tsp. allspice
1/8 tsp. black pepper
¼ cup basil
Olives (optional)

Cut the meat into individual ribs. Heat olive oil on medium high and brown ribs well on all sides. You might have to work in batches.

In the mean time, chop the onion well and place in a bowl (let's call it bowl #1). Chop the garlic and parsley. Place them in another bowl (this will be bowl #2).

Now, in a small, dry container (this will be bowl #3) put in the following spices and mix them well: bay leaf, cinnamon, cloves, allspice, black pepper. **IMPORTANT: Bowl #3 should be dry so that the spices can be mixed well.**

While the meat is browning, take a wide shallow pan (e.g. a paella pan) in which all ribs will fit without too much crowding. Heat a little olive oil and sauté chopped onion well. Add the contents of bowl #2 and sauté – stirring for another minute. Add the contents of bowl #3 and mix well.

Once the meat is browned, transfer the ribs to the paella pan and arrange in a single layer. Pour in the tomatoes and wine. Cover and let sit on low simmer for about 1.5 hours, or until the meat starts to fall off the bone.

At that point, take the ribs out. Uncover the pan. Then, increase the heat to medium high and boil well to thicken the remaining liquid (for about 15 minutes). Reduce the heat to low again, return the ribs, cover and leave them in for 5 minutes to get hot. Season with freshly chopped basil.

Serve hot immediately with ribs on the bottom, a spoon of the sauce on top, and some olives to garnish.

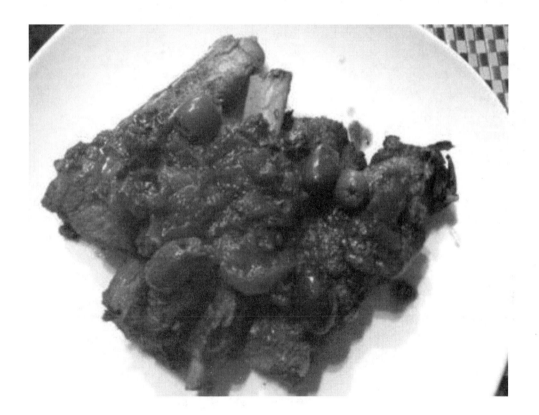

Pork Loin

This is a great recipe to make on a busy midweek evening. It's very easy. However, beware of overcooking as it will get too dry. While the loin is baking, you can cut a salad or roast some veggies.

Veggies are best roasted at 400F. However, you can still put them on the baking sheet together with the pork. They will probably not brown but will still be good. After you take the meat out, you can put the oven to broil which will brown the veggies and make them crisp.

Prep time: 3 min.   Cook time: 30 min.

Ingredients:

1 pork loin
5 garlic cloves, whole
Red wine

Place the pork into a baking pan filled with some water (about ½ inch in height) and 2-3 tbsp. of olive oil. Pour a little red wine over the pork. Next, cut 4-5 small pockets along the length of the meat (perpendicular; evenly spaced) and stuff each one with a garlic clove. Season generously all around with salt, black pepper, and oregano.

Broil for 30 minutes. Again, you have to make sure not to overcook the loin because it will get dry. You want it tender and slightly pink (keep in mind that the meat will cook a little more after you take it out of the oven).

Let it sit for a couple of minutes before cutting it into 1-inch thick slices.

Pork Chops

Of course, there are numerous ways of making chops... but here is my simple recipe.

Ingredients:

Pork chop with bone
Oregano
Lemon

Wash the meat and dry well with a paper towel. Place in an ovenproof pan. Put ample amounts of salt, black pepper, and oregano on top. Place in the oven on broil for 7-10 minutes. At that point, turn the chop over and coat that side with salt, black pepper, and oregano. Broil for another 7-10 minutes.

Cut the chop with a knife at a thick area to check how cooked it is. It will probably take you a few trials before you learn to get it just right. If you cut it and it's too raw, return to the oven and check again in another 2 minutes.

Be careful not to overcook. If it's a tad pink when you cut at the thickest part – perfect. Take the pan out of the oven and let the chop sit there for another 2-3 minutes. The meat will continue to cook just to perfection simply by sitting in the pan.

Serve with plenty of freshly squeezed lemon.

Pork With Cabbage Casserole

This recipe has two parts. First you boil the ingredients. Then, you bake them in the oven. The good news is that it is hard to get it wrong and requires very few ingredients.

Prep time: 20 min.   Cook time: 45 min. + 20 min.

Ingredients:

1-2 lbs. of any cut of pork (pork belly is best)
1 green cabbage, medium
1 tomato, chopped
1 bay leaf
Paprika
1 carrot (optional)

Chop the cabbage and sauté in oil until it becomes soft. You might have to do this in batches since the cabbage will have a lot of volume when first chopped. Add a tablespoon of paprika and the chopped tomato. Cover with hot water (add only enough water to cover it) and bring to a boil. Lower the heat and simmer for 45 minutes.

In the meantime, you can boil the meat. Wash it well, put it in water, bring to a boil, lower the heat, and let it sit on low boil until it is cooked. The cooking time will depend on the type and size of meat used (e.g. pork belly takes approximately 40 minutes). Regardless, a good rule of thumb is to boil it slowly, at low heat. You'll know it's ready when, after cutting it with a knife, it's no longer pink and/or bloody.

When cooked, take it out and allow it cool. If you used a cut with bones, separate the meat from the bones. Cut it into bite-sized pieces.

When the cabbage is done, transfer it to a casserole. However, **do not transfer all the water with the cabbage (*just enough to have half of the cabbage immersed in liquid*)**. Layer the meat bites on top and season with one bay leaf, oregano, salt, and a little more paprika. You can also grate a carrot on top at this point. Do not mix.

Place in the oven at 350 degrees for 15-20 minutes until the dish "tightens" a little (i.e. the liquid evaporates). Remember, everything is already cooked. You just want to blend all aromas together and evaporate some of the water. Serve garnished with freshly chopped parsley.

Raw Tuna Steak

Bought ready – no cooking needed.

Once in a while you may want to treat yourself to a delicious raw piece of tuna. It's expensive but so worth it. They go for $20-27 a pound and a good size steak will run you an average of $20.

You can have this instead of take-out on one of those nights when you work late or simply do not want to cook. It might seem expensive for one meal, yet, it is much better than going out to a sushi restaurant and it is as nutritious as it gets. The Japanese call this Sashimi.

IMPORTANT: Find a good local fish store that sells fresh tuna. I found mine through a Japanese friend. As it turns out, this is the place where all Japanese folks in my town go to get fresh fish to make sushi at home. **Ask the seller if the tuna is good for sushi. Do not buy unless you find a store like that**. Usually, if you live next to the coastline, you will have no problem. If not, you might have to pay more for this treat.

Wash the steak clean, pat dry and serve cold. You can add a little bit of soy sauce or wasabi. Garnish with a leaf of parsley and a lemon. You will find the raw tuna steak very filling just by itself. For sides, any fresh uncooked veggies go well.

WARNING: Your tuna (as well as any other large fish) will most likely have a high level of mercury. Unfortunately, our oceans are polluted with heavy metals and mercury poisoning is a risk for many people who eat tuna and other large fishes regularly.

The biggest danger is for pregnant women as mercury is harmful to the developing fetus. It you eat large wild caught fish regularly (once or twice a week), you need to find out about the mercury levels. This is a sad, but true, fact. Fish is one of the healthiest food choices but we must be careful.

Skirt Steak Roll

Prep time: 5 min.   Cook time: 75 min.

Ingredients:

1 skirt steak
5-7 provolone cheese deli slices
1 cup baby spinach
Meat twine

For best results, use a meat mallet and tenderize the steak well. Make sure you cover the steak with a towel or saran wrap as you are hammering because you don't want juices splashing everywhere.

Season on both sides with black pepper and oregano. Layer the cheese on top of the steak, followed by the spinach. Roll the steak along the full length. You will end up with a long roll.

Tie with the meat twine any way you like so that it doesn't fall apart during cooking.

Heat olive oil on medium high and brown the roll well on all sides. Wrap in aluminum foil and place in the preheated oven at 400F for about 30 minutes, or until the roll records 130F with a meat thermometer. This is for medium rare. Have it reach 150F if you like it medium.

Take the meat out and let it sit for an additional 5-10 minutes. Cut into ½ inch slices and serve.

Quick Leek Meat Stew

This is one of those easy, "can't go wrong" recipes. Keep in mind, the prep. time is a little longer than the other recipes because it includes the boiling of the meat (see below).

Prep time: 30 min.   Cook time: 20 min.

Ingredients:

4 leaks
1 lb. of any boneless cut of beef or pork (stew meat works good)
16 oz. chopped tomatoes (fresh or canned)

Place the meat in a boiling pot with water. Put on high heat until the water begins to boil. Then, reduce to a low simmer until the meat is cooked. This will take about 15-20 minutes depending on what cut you use (e.g. beef loin needs about 20 minutes per pound).

While the meat is cooking, chop the leeks and sauté them in olive oil on medium heat for about 7-10 minutes. Sprinkle with paprika and salt. Next, use a ladle to transfer a cup of the liquid from the boiling pot the meat is cooking in.

Once the meat is cooked, cut it into stew-sized pieces. Add it to the leeks. Next, add the tomatoes and leave for 20 minutes on low heat to get thicker. Remember, at this point everything is already cooked: the meat is boiled and the leek is sautéed. These last 20 minutes (on low heat) are essentially cooking the tomatoes and mixing all of the flavors together.

Beef Pot Roast

This is a very delicious recipe worth making once a week. It provides 6-8 servings and is very practical if you don't have the time to prepare a meal every day. It can also be made with a lamb shoulder or leg.

Prep time: 30 min.   Cook time: 2 hrs.

Ingredients:

4-5 lbs. beef chuck
1 onion
4 carrots
1 head garlic
2 cups red wine
2 cups broth (beef, chicken, or veggie)
28 oz. peeled tomatoes can (2 fresh tomatoes is even better)
½ cup fresh rosemary (or 1 tbsp. dry)
¼ cup fresh thyme (or ½ tbsp. dry)

It's best if you let the meat sit out and reach room temperature before you start (about 30-45 minutes). Wash and towel try the chuck. Sprinkle plenty of salt and black pepper on all surfaces.

Heat oil on medium high and add the meat to the oil when heated well. You need to sear the meat until brown on all surfaces. It takes about 8-10 minutes to do a thorough sear. You can cut the veggies in the meantime.

By the way, the purpose of browning the meat in hot oil is to create a surface seal to retain the moisture inside the chuck. This will prevent all the juices from leaving the meat and will create a very tender and delicious roast.

Moving on, the onion, garlic, and carrot have to be chopped. When the meat it browned on all sides, remove it and set aside. Add the vegetables in the oil and sauté for about 10 minutes on medium heat until softened and slightly browned. You might need to add some additional olive oil.

Put everything together and simmer.

Because it is better to use a pot that fits the chuck as snug as possible, it is hard to return the meat at this point. Therefore, when the vegetables are well cooked and beginning to brown, take them out, put the beef back in the pot, and cover with the vegetables, tomatoes, wine, broth, rosemary, and thyme.

You will find that the meat will not always be completely covered with liquid (this depends on what size pot you use). That's OK as long as it is at least half submerged.

Bring to a boil, reduce the heat, and simmer covered for about 2 hours. You can also transfer it all to the oven at 300F. After about an hour, turn the meat over.

When ready, remove the meat and cover well to keep warm. Bring the liquid to a high boil for about 15 minutes to make it thicker. Check to see if you need to add more salt or black pepper. Cream everything up with a soup blender (optional). Now you have a nice piece of tender roast and a delicious sauce to go with it.

If you use lamb shanks (second image below), this recipe is called Rosemary Braised Lamb Shanks. Lamb shanks are very expensive while shoulder and beef chuck taste just as good and are often on sale. If you have guests to impress, however, you might want to make this with shanks.

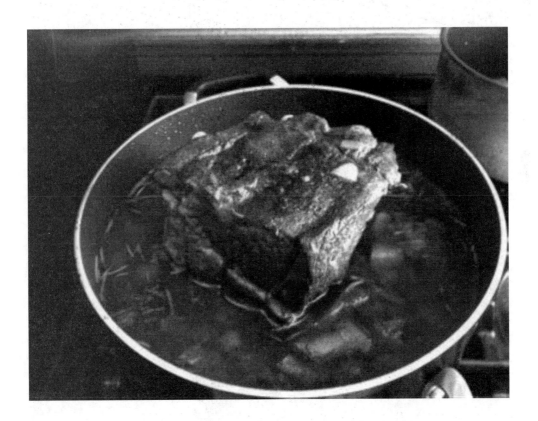

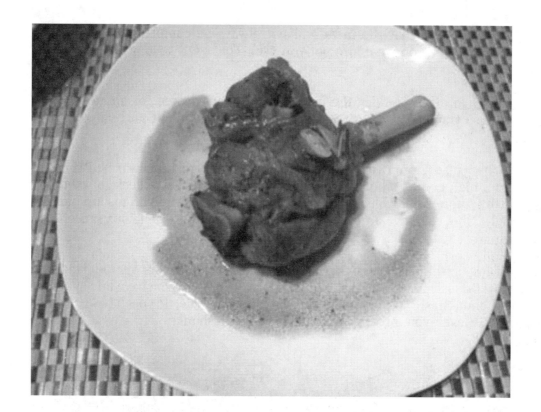

Bulgarian Patties

These are traditionally made with equal parts of ground pork and ground beef. You can change the proportions to your liking. Also, the meat will be tastier if you mix, shape them, and let them sit in the refrigerator for 2-4 hours.

Prep time: 10 min.   Cook time: 15 min.

Ingredients:

1 lb. ground beef
1 lb. ground pork
1 small onion, chopped
1 egg
½ tsp. black pepper
½ tsp. cumin
4 tsp. salt

Mix all ingredients in a large bowl. Shape the meat into patties. Flatten the center part a little bit to get somewhat a donut shape (without the hole, of course). By doing this, you make sure the middle parts cooks just as well as the outer parts.

You can cook these in all kinds of ways (e.g. oven, barbeque). The most common is to heat olive oil on medium high and brown the burgers well on both sides. The time for this varies, depending on how big they are.

Spring Lamb Steaks

This is a simple Greek recipe with a lot of color and a rich taste.

Prep Time: 30 min.   Cook time: 60 min.

Ingredients:

4 shoulder lamb steaks with the bone
1 medium onion
6 green onions
2 carrots
Juice of one lemon
1 cup of fresh peas or sugar snap peas
Fresh dill

Heat some olive oil in a pan (on medium high) and brown the chops on both sides. Set aside.

In the same oil, sauté the chopped onion, spring onions, and carrots (in that order). Be sure to wait 1-2 minutes before adding each of the above ingredients.

Bring the lamb steaks back to the pan and squeeze one full lemon directly on top of them. Give it a minute or two to evaporate. Add just enough water to cover the meat and season with salt and black pepper.

Cover and simmer on medium low heat for 45 minutes to an hour. Turn the meat over mid way.

In the last 10 minutes, add fresh peas and dill, and remove the lid.

Finally, serve with some fresh dill sprinkled on top.

Chicken in Red Wine

Prep time: 20 min.   Cook time: 2-3 hours

Ingredients:

6-8 chicken thighs
2 cups chicken or vegetable broth
2 cups dry red wine
1 onion
1 large carrot
3 garlic gloves
10 pearl onions
1 bay leaf
1 tbsp. thyme
2 tbsp. parsley

Rinse the meat and pat it dry with a paper towel. Season it on both sides with plenty of salt and black pepper. Allow thighs to reach room temperature before cooking.

In a wide pan, heat oil in medium to high heat. Brown thighs on both sides starting with the skin side down (each side takes about 8 minutes).

Transfer meat to a clean pot in which the pieces fit snuggly. It's OK to stack thighs on top of each other. Pour sliced onion, sliced carrot, peeled pearl onions, and crushed garlic gloves on top.

Pour in an equal amount of broth and wine, just enough to cover the meat. Add the bay leaf, thyme and parsley, and bring to a boil. Turn the heat down and keep at a very low simmer for about 3 hours or until the meat is so tender that it breaks apart when you put a fork or knife through it.

You can create a sauce to pour over the thighs... and you don't even need flour! When cooked, just remove the meat and bring the remaining liquid to a vigorous boil to "thicken it". After it has been boiling for about 5-10 minutes, puree it with a soup blender. Pour over the thighs and serve.

Chicken Rotisserie

Prep time: 0 min.   Cook time: 0 min.

This is one of the tastiest meals to get when you're hungry and have no time to cook. Just grab a ready roasted (preferably free-range organic) chicken and cut a quick salad on the side.

Make sure you get a plain, rosemary, or garlic chicken. Stay away from the honey glazed, barbeque, etc.... And I know what you're thinking: those are tastier. But keep in mind those sauces are also loaded with sugar.

Quick Cornish Hens

Prep time: 5 min.   Cook time: 30 min.

Ingredients:

Cornish hen
Paprika
Butter

You have several options when it comes to cooking Cornish hens. But this is one the simplest, fastest, and tastiest ways to make them. Wash and towel dry the meat. If possible, let the meat sit at room temperature for at least 30 minutes before cooking.

Cut the hen in half through the back (on the other side of the breast bone). Flatten the left and right sides and pierce two skewer sticks left to right (i.e. one through the legs and the other through the wings). The purpose of these sticks is to flatten the bird so it cooks more evenly.

Glaze all sides with butter, salt, black pepper, and paprika (paprika is the secret ingredient that gives it a simple, yet spicy, taste).

Preheat the oven at 375F, put in a baking sheet, and bake evenly on both sides for about 30 minutes total. If you prefer them crispy, put the oven to broil and leave for another 5-10 minutes to brown better.

While the bird is cooking, cut a salad or roast some veggies. Most veggies are best roasted at 400 degrees. However, they'll come out just as good if you put them alongside the meat on the baking sheet. This will get your lunch (or dinner) ready in no time.

Turkey With Cabbage

Prep time: 30 min.   Cook time: 90 min.

Ingredients:

1-2 turkey legs or 2-3 lbs. turkey meat (chopped in stew size pieces)
1 small cabbage (use any type of cabbage you like. I typically make this with regular green cabbage but sometimes mix in other types for the sake of variety)
1 large onion
1 carrot
1 leak (optional)
3 garlic cloves
Dill or parsley to garnish (optional)
Paprika

This meat is best cooked with the skin to help soften the cabbage (cabbage requires a lot of oil to cook well).

Chop the onion, garlic, carrot, and leak, and sauté well until translucent. In the meantime, chop the cabbage. You will end up with a lot of volume in a big bowl. Stir in the cabbage and sauté it as well. You might need to do this in batches since it takes up so much space initially.

Add oil as needed. A lot of olive oil will be needed to keep the cabbage from burning. This sautéing is the most time consuming part of the recipe. You can't speed it up because you will burn the cabbage. It takes a good 20 minutes to sauté everything.

Put your choice of meat in a big pot. No need for oil or spices yet. Add the sautéed ingredients on top of the meat. Add salt (I use 2 teaspoons) and 1 tablespoon of paprika. Now, add enough hot water to the pot to cover the meat.

Instead of using a lid, cover everything with a small dish (turn it upside down) and push down. This will keep the ingredients from floating to the surface of the water. At this point, the water level should be just high enough to cover the plate. No need to mix the spices and the ingredients. The water and cooking will take care of it.

Bring to a boil. Then, reduce the heat and simmer for 1.5 hours. Again, you should have just enough liquid to cover the small plate. If you put too much, the meal will turn into a soup and the taste will not be the same.

However, if that happens, don't panic. There *is* a solution. When the meat is tender and cooked, transfer everything to a casserole in the oven and broil. This will evaporate all of the excess water and brown the cabbage to a delicious taste. Alternatively, if you don't want to deal with the oven, just remove some of the excess liquid and cook a little longer under higher heat to help more of the liquid evaporate.

When finished, add some dill or parsley on top.

Now, a word of warning: This is light meal. It is not very filling as it is simply cabbage and bird. You probably won't have a hard time eating two plates in one sitting just to get full. This is why it's usually made in a big pot that accommodates large volume.

BONUS TIP: If you have a turkey farm nearby, you can stock up on frozen 2-3lb pieces of dark meat in the freezer. Dark meat is tastier and evidently much cheaper since everybody is requesting the "clean" white meat.

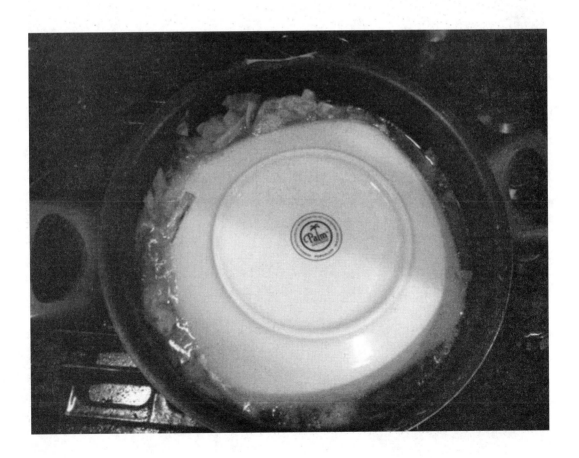

Roasted Turkey Breast

Prep time: 5 min.   Cook time: 120 min.

Ingredients:

3 lb. bone in turkey breast
½ cup chicken stock
1 lemon

Spices:

3 garlic cloves minced
2 tsp. fresh rosemary (or 1 teaspoon dry)
1 tsp. dry mustard
½ tsp. dried sage
½ tsp. dried thyme
1 tsp. salt
½ tsp. pepper
1 ½ tsp. olive oil

Preheat the oven at 325F.

Combine all spices in a bowl and mix well. Rub the mix all over the meat, even under the skin if you can reach. Place the turkey breast in a baking dish. Squeeze the juice of one lemon on top. Add the chicken stock to the pan and roast uncovered for 90-120 minutes or until the skin is darkened and the internal temperature is about 165 degrees. Let it cool for 10 minutes before you cut into it!

Asian Chicken and Shrimp

Marinade time: 60 min.   Cook time: 7 min.

Ingredients:

1 lb. skinless boneless chicken breast
12 oz. shrimps – skinned and deveined
6 shallots
6 garlic cloves
3 red hot chilies (mix different types such as regular red hot, chilies and red Thai
                bird chilies)
1 ½ inch piece of ginger
½ lime

Chop the chilies, shallots and garlic. Grate the ginger. Place all in a food processor (if you have one, otherwise mince everything as small as you can). Add 1 tablespoon of olive oil and 1 teaspoon of salt.

Cut the chicken breast into bite-sized pieces, place the shrimp next to it and add 2 tablespoons of the mixture you just made. Spread the mixture on top but do not mix the chicken and shrimp as they will be cooked separately. Cover and refrigerate for 1 hour.

Heat 2 tablespoons of olive oil in a skillet over medium heat. Place the remaining marinade and cook stirring regularly for about 5 minutes.

Add the chicken to the pan, increase the heat to medium-high, and cook for 2 minutes. Add the shrimp and cook for another 3-4 minutes. Season with salt to taste and serve immediately.

Rich Thai Chicken With Greens

Ever wonder how those Asian restaurants serve meals that taste so exotic? Well, you need a lot of ingredients to make a recipe like this. If you like Asian food, it is worth buying a jar of Thai curry and fish sauce because you will want to make this again. I suggest making this on a Friday or Saturday night at home. It would almost be like going out to a restaurant, except, it is all healthy and will not count as a cheat meal.

Prep time: 5 min.   Cook time: 30 min.

Ingredients:

1 lb. boneless chicken breast, cut into large pieces
1 lb. oyster mushrooms
3 garlic cloves
1 ½ tbsp. red curry paste
1 cup chicken broth
13 oz. coconut milk
3 cups snap peas
1 tbsp. fish sauce

Greens for topping:

1 cup bean sprouts
½ cup watercress
½ cup cilantro
2 scallions
1 jalapeno
½ lime

You will need a large frying pan. Now, this is a fast moving recipe so it's a good idea to have all your ingredients ready to go. Have the following clean and ready:

- Mushrooms
- Chopped garlic
- Snap peas
- Beansprouts, watercress, cilantro, scallions, jalapeño, lime juice – all in one bowl

Heat 3-4 tablespoons of olive oil until it starts to smoke. Add the mushrooms and season with salt and pepper. Cook for 2-3 minutes and lower the heat to medium.

Add the garlic – cook for 30 seconds stirring the whole time.

Next, add the curry paste. That also stays in for 30 seconds with constant stirring.

Now, add the broth and coconut milk. Let these heat up and start to simmer.

Add the chicken and adjust the heat as needed to maintain the simmering for about 20 minutes. At about minute 10, turn the chicken upside down. When cooked, take the chicken out on a plate and let it sit to cool.

Reduce the heat to low and add the snap peas. When the chicken is cool enough to handle, cut into pieces with your hand and introduce back in the pan. Cook for another 2 minutes to get the snap peas cooked but still crispy. Add half of the fish sauce.

Now, you are done!

Asian Chicken With Green Beans

Love Asian food but don't want to eat the unhealthy foods that come with the meals in some Asian restaurants? Here is how to make a tasty Asian recipe at home and save some money too.

Prep time: 5 min.   Cook time: 5 min.

Ingredients:

½ boneless, skinless chicken breasts, cut into thin slices
2 tbsp. Thai red curry paste
¼ lb. green beans
1 tbsp. fish sauce
1 tbsp. oyster sauce

Heat olive oil in a large frying pan on medium-high. Add the 2 tbsp. of curry paste and stir well for a bout 30 seconds, pressing down at the pan to incorporate the paste well into the oil.

Add the green beans and put the heat on high. From now on, keep stirring until the end.

Cook the beans for 1 minute. Then, add the chicken, the fish, and oyster sauces. Keep stirring until the chicken is cooked (another 1-2 minutes). At the end, you can try the sauce and add more fish sauce or more water, depending on your taste.

Serve immediately.

Plain Chicken With Any Seasoning

This is the simplest and quickest way to cook a whole chicken to delicious crispness and with full moisture retained.

Prep time: 5 min.   Cook time: 50 min.

Ingredients:

1 whole chicken
Roasting pan
Aluminum foil
Butter (olive oil is OK too)
Garlic, rosemary, salt, pepper (or other spices or spice mix of your choice)

Preheat oven at 500F.

Blot the chicken dry with paper towels as much as possible. If you dry it really well, you will get a crispier chicken.

Melt some butter between your palms and spread all over. Alternatively, coat well with olive oil. This coating seals the moisture inside the chicken so it doesn't dry up during cooking.

Finally, mince the garlic and spread evenly over the bird together with the rest of the spices used – salt, pepper, paprika, garlic salt, etc.

Take a sheet of aluminum foil, about the size of half of your baking dish, and fold it several times over to form a triangle. Don't go crazy with the details here. Just make it into a triangular shape of aluminum foil, large enough to cover the breast. Now, this triangle should not be one sheet thick but about 3 sheets thick or more to work well.

Place the chicken in the baking dish with the chest up, cover the breast with the aluminum, and place in the oven for 20 minutes. The purpose of the aluminum is to keep the breast from overcooking and turning dry.

After 20 minutes, you will see the legs begin the brown. Remove the aluminum and continue to cook it at 500F for another 30 minutes.

Important: when finished, take it out of the oven and let it sit for 10-15 minutes. This step is essential. If you start cutting into it sooner, all the moisture on the inside will flow out and your chicken will taste dry. Let it sit for a good 15 minutes and the inside juices will redistribute and settle leaving you with a tender chicken.

Chicken Breast With Zucchini And Carrots

Prep time: 10 min.   Cook time: 50 min.

Ingredients:

4 tbsp. olive oil
2 lemons
4 cloves garlic
1 tsp. salt
½ tsp. black pepper
2 zucchini
4 large carrots, chopped in large pieces
2 chicken breasts (bones left in, with skin)

Preheat oven to 400°F.

Coat a baking dish with olive oil. Cut one of the lemons into slices and arrange them in a single layer at the bottom.

In a large bowl, put 4 tablespoons of olive oil, squeeze the juice of the second lemon, mince the garlic and put in with the salt and the pepper. Mix well.

Slice the zucchini in circles, toss in the oil mix and coat well. Place the zucchini on top of the lemon slices (use a slotted spoon to take them out and save the spiced olive oil in the bowl). Repeat the same with the carrots and place them on top of the zucchini.

Place the chicken in the bowl and coat well. Position the chicken on top of the carrots with the skin up and pour the remaining spiced olive oil on op.

Cook uncovered for 50 minutes.

Fish and Seafood

Seafood is one of the best things you can eat. It's a great source of protein and essential heart-healthy fats (e.g. omega-3's). That said, if you don't like it (or you're allergic to fish or seafood) you don't have to eat it.

Remember, The Cruise Control Diet is very flexible and adaptable to each individual's lifestyle. However, if you're a fan of the "fruits of the sea", try these recipes and feel free to explore more of your own.

Simply Delicious Fish Soup

Back in the day, fish soup was considered a cheap daily meal that everyone was bored of. It was cheap because it was made with the left over pieces of all kinds of fish. As such, you can use any type of fish to make this. In fact, you should mix 2-3 different types for a richer taste. Just cut the pieces into large bite-sized chunks.

Prep time: 5 min.   Cook time: 15 min.

Ingredients:

1.5 lbs. fish fillet
1 onion (chopped)
2 garlic gloves (chopped)
Parsley
1 medium tomato (chopped)
2 tsp. tomato paste
8 oz. clam juice (or shellfish stock)
2/3 cup white wine
Thyme
Oregano

Sauté the onion and garlic on medium heat in olive oil. After 4 minutes, add the parsley, stir and leave in for another 2 minutes. Next, add the chopped tomato and tomato paste and leave in for 2 more minutes.

Add in the fish, wine, clam juice, and continue to simmer for about 5-8 minutes, until the fish is cooked. Depending on the type of fish, this might take a few minutes longer. Just make sure you are simmering and not boiling.

Season with a pinch of oregano, thyme, fresh parsley, salt, and black pepper to taste. Serve hot.

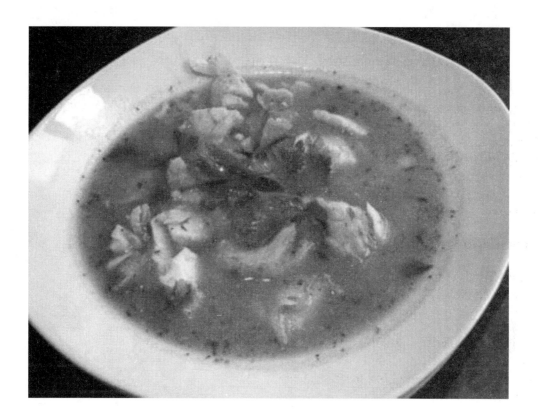

Mark's Five Minute Recipe For Fish

Mark and Fiona are two followers of The Cruise Control Diet who are also very good chefs. They were happy to share one of their own recipes with the other readers. Thank you Fiona and Mike!

Prep time: 5 min.   Cook time: 20 min.

Ingredients:

4 white fish fillets
2 tbsp. coconut oil
13 oz. coconut milk
2 tsp. turmeric powder (or more to taste)
2 garlic cloves
1 chili pepper
2 spring onions
½ red onion
2 carrots
2 tsp. turmeric

Chop the garlic, red onion and chili, and place them in bowl #1. Grind the carrot and place in bowl #2.

Combine coconut oil with a little salt, chopped garlic, onion and chili, and fry gently until the onion is transparent. Add coconut milk and turmeric and stir.

Add the fish fillets, grated carrot, and whatever other vegetables such as sliced zucchini, snow peas, or bean sprouts that you might have.

Cook together gently on medium low until fish is cooked. Depending on the type of fish this could be 10-20 minutes. You can add some fish or vegetable stock to moisten.

Serve with chopped spring onions to garnish.

Note: The original recipe was with coconut cream. This can be one of those hidden sources of sugar that you should avoid. Some brands have 20 grams of sugar in 2 tablespoons. One full can is 15 times that amount. It is better to use milk unless you can find no-sugar added coconut cream.

Italian Fish and Seafood Stew

Did you know that some of the more impressive classic old world recipes are also the easiest to make? No need to go to the Italian restaurant to get something gourmet in you house. This one is a real gem.

Basically, you make a lot of this broth and you freeze it packaged in servings. When ready to eat, take some broth out, heat it up, throw in any fish or seafood you want for no more than a few minutes, and eat while hot. There is nothing better than a homemade warm stew that is ready in minutes. Here is how to make the broth:

Prep time: 5 min.   Cook time: 30 min.

Ingredients:

¾ cup butter
2 onions
2 garlic cloves
25 oz. crushed tomatoes
64 oz. broth of your choice (fish stock is ideal, clam juice can be used too)
1 ½ cup white wine

Spices (fresh for best results, can be dried):

2 bay leaves
1 tbsp. basil
½ tsp. thyme
½ tsp. oregano

Start by chopping the onion, garlic, and parsley. Melt the butter in the large pot and add the chopped onion, garlic, and parsley. Let them mix well and soften. Stir from time to time and keep at medium-low heat.

When softened, pour in the rest of the ingredients. Put them all in, add a cup of water, and mix well. Bring to a boil and let simmer for 30 min. That's it!

This will make you a large amount of stock. Let it cool and freeze separated into smaller portions. When ready with some seafood, reheat the stock, add to it whatever you like – any type of fish, shrimp, mussels, crabs, scallops, clams, etc.. The more different items you mix, the better it comes out. Cook for a few minutes only at medium heat.

Sprinkle with fresh parsley to impress and serve hot.

Halibut Filets

This is a light meal – great for lunch. If you are a big eater, double the recipe.

Prep time: 10 min.   Cook time: 15 min.

Ingredients:

2 halibut filets
2 tbsp. pesto
1 carrot
½ zucchini
2 tsp. white wine
Olive oil, salt, pepper
Butter
Parchment paper

Preheat oven to 450F. Shred the carrot and zucchini.

Prepare parchment paper by following these instructions: Start with a rectangular (12 x 18 or large rectangle) parchment paper. Fold in half, just like a book closes. Draw a large half heart (something like a huge question mark). Cut with scissors along the line you just drew and open up the "book" – now you should have parchment paper in the shape of a large heart.

You need a heart for each filet.

Place a little butter only on one side of the heart (about a teaspoon). Be careful not to put any butter around the edges or on the other side. In fact, stay well clear of the edges.

 Rinse the filets in cold water and pat dry. Place a filet over the butter followed by a tablespoon of pesto, half of the shredded carrot, and half the shredded zucchini. Add salt and pepper to taste. Dazzle with a teaspoon of wine and a teaspoon of olive oil.

Close the heart (like a book again). Make small, tight, and overlapping folds along the parchment edges to create an airtight seal. Start with the top and close tightly at the bottom of the heart.

Bake for 15 minutes.

Mango Salmon in Parchment Paper

There are literally endless combinations of fish, veggies, and fruits that can be cooked using the heart shaped parchment paper described in the previous recipe. Here is another favorite.

Prep time: 10 min.   Cook time: 15 min.

Ingredients:

2 salmon filets
½ small onion
1 ripe mango
1 chili pepper
2 tsp. white wine
Olive oil, salt, pepper
Butter
Parchment paper

Preheat oven to 450F.

Prepare the parchment hearts as in the previous recipe. Place the butter followed by the pat dried salmon. Follow with chopped onion and chili pepper. Cut a ripe mango in long thin (French fries looking) strips. Place these on top. Season with salt and pepper and toss with olive oil and white wine.

Fold the hearts, seal the outline with overlapping folds, and bake for 15 minutes.

Crab Stuffed Fish Filet

Crabmeat is easy to find here in New England. You only need a spoonful for this quick recipe. A good choice for cheese is one of those already flavored cheese spreads like cheese with roasted pepper, cheese with chive, etc.

Prep time: 5 min.   Cook time: 15 min.

Ingredients:

2 fish filets (flounder, tilapia, cod, anything flat that is easy to roll)
2 tbsp. of crabmeat
2 tbsp. cheese of your choice
1 lemon

Preheat oven to 350F.

Mix the crabmeat with the cheese. Add two spoonfuls of the mixture in the middle of the filet (where it is widest) and roll each end on top to make a roll.

Bake for 15 minutes.

Serve with freshly squeezed lemon juice. You could garnish with chopped parsley or chives.

E. Breakfast Ideas

After you eliminate starchy carbs and sugars from your diet, you won't be waking up starving and rushing to put something in your mouth.

And by something, I mean a bagel, donut, muffin, cereal, sandwich, etc. All of this topped with an OJ sugar injection. Come to think of it, are there any breakfast foods *not* loaded with sugar?

Now, as shocking as this may sound to many people (hopefully not to you anymore), bacon and eggs is one of the healthiest breakfasts you can have. Ideally, you should eat only cage-free organic eggs and bacon with no preservatives or nitrates.

I'm sure you have your own favorite way of making eggs. But here are a couple more worth trying (plus some egg-free ideas).

Pepper Feta Omelet

This is a version of the classic combination of eggs, peppers, and feta cheese. It is very quick to make. Now, if you prefer larger servings, add more eggs but remember to add more peppers as well. The ideal ratio is 4:1 (eggs to peppers; e.g. 2 eggs for ½ pepper; 4 eggs for 1 pepper, etc.…). The amount of feta may vary based on your taste preferences.

Ingredients:

1/2 red bell pepper (any color will do)
2 eggs
1 tomato
2 tbsp. of feta cheese

Chop the pepper into bite size chunks and sauté it in olive oil or butter on medium low heat until it starts to brown. Crumble the feta on top. Chop the tomato well and put it in. This will make the mix watery and it will start to boil. Add a little more water (e.g. a tbsp.) if needed. Beat the eggs with a little salt and add them last. Mix well. As soon as the eggs cook (approx. 2 minutes), your meal is ready.

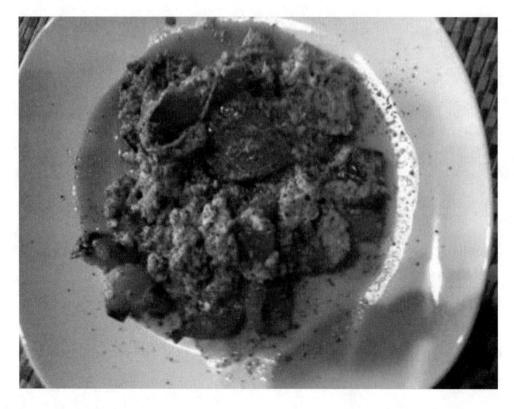

Peppers Stuffed with Eggs and Feta Cheese

This breakfast can be prepared in advance and reheated later or even eaten cold.

Prep time: 35 min. (or 5 min.)   Cook time: 30 min.

Ingredients:

5 eggs
1 cup feta cheese
3 red bell peppers
28 oz. chopped tomatoes can *or*...
1 fresh tomato and 1 cup of tomato sauce

Preheat the oven at 400F and roast the bell peppers until they brown on all sides (about 30 minutes). Wrap with a paper towel and let them "suffocate" and cool. When cooled enough to handle, peel the skins and chop the stems off.

If you're short on time, you could also get peppers that are already roasted and cut your prep time to just 5 minutes.

Beat the eggs well and mix with the feta cheese. Season with a little black pepper. Take a spoon and fill each pepper with this mix.

Next, take a small ceramic dish (just big enough to hold all the peppers) and line the bottom of it with a little olive oil... just enough so that the peppers don't stick. You can put a few drops on there and spread it out with your fingers.

Cover the stuffed peppers with the chopped tomato, and pour the tomato sauce. Place in the oven at 350F for about 30 minutes... or until the sauce boils well.

You can garnish with fresh chopped parsley and serve immediately or eat them cold later.

Finally, as you may have noticed, we didn't use salt in this recipe. The feta is already salty enough and that will transfer over to the rest of the stuffing. However, if you use a fresh tomato (instead of canned) you can sprinkle the stuffed peppers with a little salt before baking them.

Nuts and Apples

This is a very filling "breakfast to go". Raw, unsalted almonds are my nuts of choice but any other will do (e.g. walnuts, hazelnuts). This meal will keep you full for hours. A good proportion is 2/3 cup of almonds and one apple. Also, you don't need to cut the apple and mix it with the nuts. Just eat it as is and pop some almonds in between.

Yogurt with Walnuts

Prep time: 2 min.   Cook time: 0 min.

This is more of a treat than a meal as it is best to limit dairy somewhat. It can be eaten as a breakfast about once a week. It is really tasty if you add some berries.

Make sure the yogurt is whole milk and plain: no added flavors or fruits. Only full fat, whole, plain yogurt. Crumble some walnuts on top. Add your choice of berries.

You can experiment with this any way you like. Try almonds instead of walnuts. Just don't put anything sugary in there like raisins and other dried fruits.

Carrots, Pickle, Egg

This is a good breakfast if you don't want to eat a heavy meal in the morning but, at the same time, don't want to start the day on an empty stomach. The quantities given are for a small breakfast, about 200 calories. Feel free to add more carrots or eggs as needed.

Ingredients:

2 boiled carrots
2 boiled eggs
1 pickle

The secret to most meals is presentation. Slice the egg in circles and spice with salt, pepper, and paprika. Arrange the carrot and pickle next to it. This can be prepared ahead of time and grabbed in the morning as a snack at work.

Two Avocados

Avocados are one of those super foods that can be eaten as is, without cooking. They are very caloric and will fill you up until lunchtime. In fact, two avocados provide about 500 calories. Remember, the reason I am giving you the calories is not because we are looking for low calorie breakfasts. Just the opposite: we want a lot of good calories that will satisfy you and give you the energy to go through your day.

How to choose avocados:

Avocados are ready to eat when the center feels firm but the two ends are starting to get soft. If the whole fruit feels soft, it's too late. It will taste overripe and won't be edible. If the ends are not slightly soft, it needs a day or two more to ripen. When you buy avocados, choose the ones that are firm and let them ripen at home.

How to eat the avocado:

Take a knife and cut the fruit in half ending with two long halves, one of which will contain the pit. Scoop out the pit with a spoon. Scoop and eat the avocado straight from the shell with the spoon.

Smoked Fish

Some love it – others hate it. If you are one of those people that does like smoked fish, why not have it at breakfast?!

Ingredients:

Smoked fish of your choice
1 small cucumber
1 ripe tomato
1 slice of feta
4-5 olives

Simply serve yourself a piece of smoked fish of your choice and garnish with the rest of the ingredients. You can sprinkle the feta and tomatoes with olive oil along with a bit of salt and oregano.

Baked Acorn Squash with Cinnamon

This recipe is ideal for people with a sweet tooth or those who are used to having a sweet every morning. Acorn squash has a natural sweetness that won't interfere with your weight loss and cinnamon is one of those spices that actually accelerate weight loss.

Ingredients:

1 whole acorn squash
Cinnamon

Preheat the oven at 400F.

Cut the squash in two, scoop out the seeds and place in a baking pan with the cut side facing up. Add about ¼ inch of water to the pan to prevent the skin from drying. Bake for about 1 hour and 15 minutes or until the squash can easily be penetrated with a fork.

Take out and sprinkle with cinnamon. Allow to cool. Eat directly with a spoon.

Any type of squash or pumpkin can be used in this recipe. The only thing that might vary is the cooking time. Just check with your fork from time to time to see if it's ready.

Now, who has an hour to prepare breakfast, right? You can bake this in advance and have it ready to go. It can be reheated.

Non-Grain "Cereal"

Nuts and seeds are excellent sources of important nutrients. Why not start the day with them? This recipe is for those hard-core cereal breakfast eaters. Instead of cereal, fill you bowl with any or all of the following:

- Pumpkin seeds
- Sunflower seeds
- Flaxseeds
- Sliced almonds
- Berries

Try that with whole milk, almond, or coconut milk (make sure you buy a brand that is natural and does not have added sugars). Note: do not be tempted to put dried fruits like raisins. These are not a good way to start the day as they have too much sugar. Stick with fresh berries or apple slices. Stay away from bananas as well.

The Cruise
Control Diet
JUMPSTART GUIDE

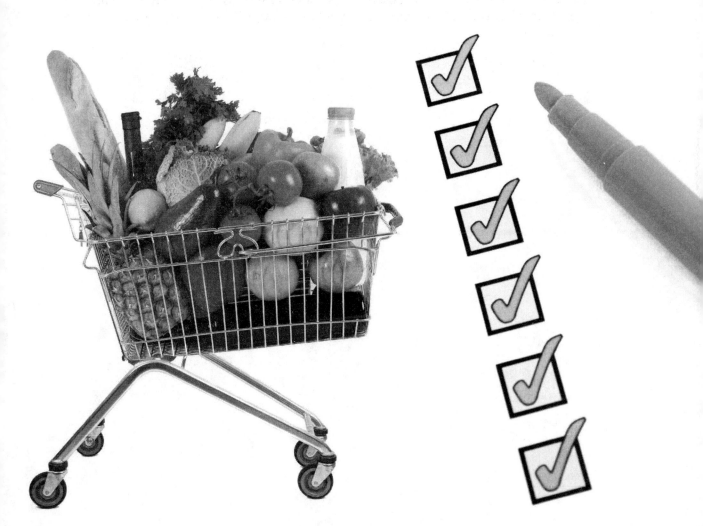

JAMES WARD

A Short Intro to This Guide...

The Cruise Control Diet is meant to be a very loose program. It doesn't bog you down with the many rules and restrictions that come with most other diets. And that's the secret behind its success. You can stay on it for the long run and essentially break that dreaded cycle of losing and regaining the same 5, 10, or 20 pounds.

For the most part, you just eat the foods that promote fat loss (and ultimately health) while avoiding the ones that prevent it. And once you know what these are... your meal plans are limited only by your imagination. There are literally endless amounts of food combinations available to you.

With that said, some people prefer to have a bit of structure and guidance... especially when getting started. And if you happen to be in that camp, this short guide will help you transition smoothly into the Cruise Control Diet's eating plan.

Now, before I lay it out for you, I'd like to make you aware of the following:

1) This is just a rough outline; you don't need to follow it to the "T". In fact, if you're good with grocery shopping (and cooking in general) you can even skip it altogether.

2) After putting everything in words, I realize that I eat a lot of food (a TON actually). You might be smaller in size and need less food to get by. That's fine; simply adjust the portions accordingly.

3) The grocery shopping list and meal plans are for a single person (who eats a LOT). If you're feeding a family of two, four, etc. – again – adjust the amounts accordingly.

4) I'm assuming that you're a busy person with a job you go to on most days of the week. As such, I've listed some of the most basic meals you can put together. This will help you out if you're new to the "sport" of cooking.

   But, once you get better at it, you can dive into some of the more complex (and tastier) recipes found in the cook book.

5) Continuing with the point above, I've structured your meals in a way in which you'll be cooking a double portion for your dinners so that you have leftovers to take to work for lunch on the following day.

6) Finally, I have also included a section of meal plans for people who can't cook due to certain restrictions (e.g. no time, assisted living, etc.).

Please note: this is NOT the best way to eat as far as your health is concerned because it requires you to buy pre-packaged foods. Furthermore, nothing will give you better weight loss results than preparing your own meals.

That said, some people really can't cook for whatever reason. And if this describes you, the alternate meal plans provide you with a compromise that will still give you great results.

Alright, let's dive in. We'll start with the meals you prepare yourself...

Your Grocery Shopping List

OK, let's take a trip to the supermarket. We're going to stock up on a week's worth of food. Remember to adjust quantities if you're shopping for your spouse, partner, family, etc...

We'll start with the meats and fish:

(1) Pork loin

(4) Hamburger patties (fresh, not frozen)

(2) Pork chops, center-cut (with or without the bone). IMPORTANT: You will be eating this on Friday. In order to ensure it doesn't go bad, either buy it frozen or make another trip to the market later in the week (e.g. Thursday/Friday) to get it then

(6-12) Chicken drumsticks (this number will vary based on how much you normally eat. You want to get enough for two servings as you'll be eating them for a dinner and a lunch)

(2) Sausage of your preference (chicken, turkey, pork)

(1) Salmon filet (preferably wild caught)

(1) Steak (T-bone, Ribeye, etc.; ideally you should be purchasing grass-fed meat. However, I understand that pricing and availability can make this impossible for some. If this is your case, choose a leaner cut of meat; the reason why is explained in detail inside the main book). IMPORTANT: You will be eating this on Saturday. In order to ensure it doesn't go bad, either buy it frozen or make another trip to the market later in the week (e.g. Thursday/Friday) to get it then

(1) Ready cooked, rotisserie chicken (either choose the plain type, the garlic & herb, or even lemon; stay away from the BBQ and Teriyaki ones as those sauces are loaded with sugar)

Now, let's go get some veggies:

(2) Heads of Romaine lettuce

(1) Small head of green cabbage

(4) Small cucumbers

(1) Carrot (if you can't find singles, get a bag as you'll use them in the following weeks)

(1) Cauliflower

(2) Tomatoes

(3) Green bell peppers

(1) Red bell pepper

(1) Yellow or orange bell pepper

(2) Portabella mushroom caps

(1 lb.) Brussels sprouts

(1) Head of broccoli

(1) Bunch (or bag) of baby spinach

(7) Lemons

You'll need the following spices (which you probably already have): salt, pepper, and oregano.

You'll also need olive oil (extra virgin) and red wine vinegar for your salads.

Now, all we're left with are some eggs, fruits, and nuts.

Go grab a dozen eggs (or two dozen if you eat them by the bunch like I do). Any kind will do (white/brown) but ideally you'll choose the cage-free ones from chickens that were raised without antibiotics.

For fruit, I'd choose 5 apples and a box of blueberries. The latter can sometimes be hard to find (and prohibitively expensive) so if that's the case, just buy a couple more apples so you can have a piece of fruit per day.

As for nuts... a pound of raw, unsalted almonds will do just fine.

One more thing, you'll need some aluminum foil for one of the recipes so if you don't already have some, now's the time to grab it.

And that's it. You should be in and out of the supermarket in no time flat. Now let's actually plan your next week's meals.

Your Week's Meal Plans

As I put this guide together, I'm assuming you're shopping on your day off from work. I'm also assuming that this day is a Sunday. However, if it's not, I want you to use Sunday's meal plan as your first day... whatever it may be.

The reason for this is because I had you buy a ready chicken. This will be your first meal (lunch) after coming home from the grocery store. I tend to build up an appetite when I'm shopping for food and I don't have the patience to cook when I get home. A ready chicken solves that problem.

But again, this is only a rough guide. Feel free to adjust accordingly to suit your own schedule.

Now, you'll notice that I haven't included breakfast. As mentioned in the main book, I only eat breakfast about three times per week on days that I lift weights (it's always a 4-5 egg omelet with 4-5 strips of bacon). I'm just not hungry otherwise because I eat a ton of food for lunch and dinner (as you'll see below).

With that said, you might be starving in the morning (not likely after eating this way for about a week, but possible). If that's the case, feel free to eat eggs and bacon, or some fruit with nuts for your breakfast. It doesn't really matter as long as you avoid the typical "fat traps" such as cereal, pancakes, bagels, and other sugar-laden foods.

Onward...

Sunday (Shopping Day)

For Lunch:

Half of the rotisserie chicken (you will store the other half in the refrigerator for tomorrow's lunch)

Romaine lettuce salad with cauliflower bits (½ head of Romaine lettuce, 1 small cucumber, ½ green bell pepper, ¼ head cauliflower cut into pieces; add olive oil and vinegar, salt, pepper, and oregano for salad dressing)

For Dinner:

Salmon filet (see the next section for cooking instructions)

Cauliflower salad (½ head; cut the cauliflower into small pieces, pour some olive on them, and squeeze half of a fresh lemon on top. Stir well so that the oil and lemon mix with the cauliflower)

Monday

For Lunch:

Half of the rotisserie chicken (from yesterday)

Romaine lettuce salad (½ head, 1 small cucumber, ½ green bell pepper; add olive oil and vinegar, salt, pepper, and oregano for salad dressing)

For Dinner:

½ Pork Loin (see the "Meats" section on the main book for cooking instructions; you will cook the entire loin but store half of it in the refrigerator for tomorrow's lunch)

Pepper Salad (½ red bell pepper, ½ yellow bell pepper, ½ green bell pepper, 1 portabella mushroom cap; add olive oil and vinegar, salt, pepper, and oregano for salad dressing)

Tuesday

For Lunch:

½ Pork Loin (from yesterday)

Romaine lettuce salad with cauliflower bits (½ head of Romaine lettuce, 1 small cucumber, ½ green bell pepper, ¼ head cauliflower cut into pieces; add olive oil and vinegar, salt, pepper, and oregano for salad dressing)

For Dinner:

2 Burger patties (see the next section for cooking instructions; you will cook all four that you bought but store half of them in the refrigerator for tomorrow's lunch)

½ lb. Brussels sprouts (refer to the "Vegetable Side Dishes" section in the main book for cooking instructions; you will cook the entire pound that you purchased and save the other half for tomorrow's lunch)

Wednesday

For Lunch:

2 Burger patties (from yesterday)

½ lb. Brussels sprouts (from yesterday)

For Dinner:

Sausage

Cabbage salad (refer to the "Salads" section of the main book for preparation instructions)

Thursday

For Lunch:

Tuna Salad

For Dinner:

Half of the Chicken drumsticks (i.e. 3-6; see the next section for cooking instructions)

Pepper Salad (½ red bell pepper, ½ yellow bell pepper, ½ green bell pepper, 1 portabella mushroom cap; add olive oil and vinegar, salt, pepper, and oregano for salad dressing)

Friday

For Lunch:

Half of the Chicken drumsticks (i.e. 3-6 from yesterday)

Romaine lettuce salad with baby spinach leaves (½ head of Romaine lettuce, 1 small cucumber, ½ green bell pepper, handful of baby spinach leaves; add olive oil and vinegar, salt, pepper, and oregano for salad dressing)

For Dinner:

1 Pork chop (see the "Meats" section in the main book for cooking instructions; cook both chops and save one for tomorrow's lunch)

Broccoli florets (see the "Vegetable Side Dishes" section in the main book for preparation instructions)

Saturday

For Lunch:

1 Pork chop (from yesterday)

Tomato Salad (see the "Salads" section in the main book for preparation instructions)

For Dinner:

Steak (see the next section for preparation instructions)

Cabbage Dill Salad (see the "Salads" section in the main book for preparation instructions)

Now, before we move on to the actual recipes I want to give you another helpful hint. You should prepare your next day's lunch side (i.e. your salad) while you're cooking the night's dinner.

Simply cut the vegetables, put them in some kind of container, and store them in the refrigerator **without adding the salad dressing**. Otherwise, they'll be soggy (and quite nasty) by the time you sit down for lunch.

Then, you just mix the oil and vinegar or oil and lemon into another container (e.g. en empty water bottle) and add the spices if called for in the recipe (e.g. salt, pepper, oregano).

Once you're ready to eat lunch, pour your homemade dressing into your salad and you're good to go. Bon appetite!

Recipes

Salmon

This is a very easy meal to prepare. It's also fast (won't take you more than 10-15 minutes). Simply coat a broiling pan with a bit of olive oil so the fish doesn't stick. Wash and towel-dry the filet and place it in the oven to **broil** for 10, 15 minutes max.

The actual time will depend on its thickness. However, the best way to know if it's ready is to cut through it once 10 minutes have passed. The color should be light pink. If it's still dark, leave it in for a few more minutes then cut into it at a different point to examine its color.

Once cooked, squeeze the juice of half a lemon on it and you're ready to eat. Add a sprinkle of salt to your liking (optional as the lemon gives it all the taste it needs).

Burger Patties

This is another quick and easy meal to prepare. Place the patties on a broiling pan (coat it with a little oil to prevent sticking) and place it in the oven on **broil** for 10-20 minutes.

If you like your meat rare, broil the patties for 10 minutes while flipping them over halfway through. If you like your meat well done let them sit in there for closer to 20 minutes (while again, flipping them over around the 10-minute mark).

Once ready, remove them from the oven and add salt and pepper to taste. For extra flavor place a slice of American (or cheddar cheese) on each patty immediately after taking them out of the oven (the cheese will melt on the burgers while they're still hot making for a delicious meal).

Steak

Your steak can be prepared in the exact way as the patties above (same timeframe as well). The only difference being is that I don't usually coat the broiling pan with oil. The steak tends to have enough moisture so as to not stick to the pan.

One more difference with the patties: aside from salt and pepper, oregano is a third spice which will give your steak added flavor (oh yeah, and skip the cheese). Finally, you should add the spices only *after* it is cooked because the salt tends to dehydrate the meat making it less juicy.

Chicken Drumsticks

Preheat your oven to 350F. Fill a deep baking pan with a ½ inch of water. Add 3 tablespoons of olive oil and rock the pan a bit to mix the oil with the water.

Skin and wash the drumsticks and place them in the pan. Next, squeeze the juice of three lemons all over the drumsticks (use only 1 ½ lemon if cooking 6 drumsticks). Now, this is optional but for an even richer flavor, pour ½ cup of red wine over them as well.

Next, spice the meat with salt, pepper, and oregano (use generous portions of the latter). Finally, cover the pan with aluminum foil (wrap it around the edges to make it air tight) and place it in the oven. It should rest on a lower rack – just one above the absolute lowest.

Let it cook for 45 minutes. Remove the pan from the oven, take off the aluminum foil, and make sure there is enough liquid in the pan. If there is very little, add a bit of water to bring it back up to the ½ inch level. Otherwise, place the pan back in the oven for another 45 minutes. Your drumsticks will be ready after an hour and a half of total cooking time.

TIP: if you've never made something like this before, you'd be well served to check the liquid/water level at the 1 hour, and 1:15 marks to make sure it hasn't fully evaporated. The drumsticks will end up burning on the bottom if this happens so add more water if necessary.

Zero Cooking Zone

So, what about people who have no kitchen? Or don't have time to cook at all? I'm talking about busy individuals who prefer to spend as little time as possible on meal preparation. Can you eat ready-made food every day and still lose weight?

You bet! And this section will show you how.

But, as mentioned previously, I don't recommend you eat this way unless it's absolutely necessary. Nothing beats a home-cooked meal when it comes to health and weight loss. That said, there are some frozen and pre-packaged foods that are actually quite good. The trick is knowing which ones.

So, here is a week of such meals along with a grocery shopping list for you to start on Sunday.

Your Grocery Shopping List

This meal plan assumes that you'll be shopping on a Sunday afternoon before dinner and after lunch. Therefore, you will notice that the first meal listed below is dinner on Sunday night. Feel free to adjust this plan based on the day you decide to go to the grocery store.

Now, depending on the supermarket, the items available will vary a bit. Unlike the regular week of meal plans at the beginning of the Jumpstart Guide, this list will need to be modified based on what is available to you.

Fresh Veggies:

(3) Tomatoes

(2) Apples

(2) Bags of coleslaw, prewashed

> *Some stores have ready to go, made-in-store coleslaw in a container. If yours has that, check the expiration date and if it's good for at least another 4 days you can get this instead of the bagged one. Also, get this only if it doesn't have potatoes – otherwise, get the bagged one.*

(2) Bags of green salad of your choice (lettuce, baby greens, etc.), prewashed

(2) Cucumbers (or a single long one)

(1) Sweet potato

(1) Fresh vegetable platter (boxed, prewashed)

Frozen Veggies:

(1) Brussels sprouts

(2) Frozen veggie bags (your choice); Get enough for 5 salads

Frozen Meat and Dinners:

(1) Small bag of frozen, cooked shrimp

(3) Bags of meatballs, fully cooked (only buy the kind that has no pasta or anything else but the meatball)

(2) Bags of chicken, fully cooked (again, choose the ones that have no added pasta or rice. Also, make sure the chicken is not breaded)

(1) Box of beef patties, fully cooked

(1) Salmon, fully cooked or with microwave instructions

Other Items:

(½ lb.) Ham, no nitrates added (enough for 2 breakfasts)

(12) Eggs (if you don't want to boil them, buy 5 already boiled eggs)

(1) Package of bacon

(1) Jar of pickles

(½ lb.) Smoked turkey

(2) Salad dressings (one that goes well with green salad and one that goes well with coleslaw if you didn't buy the ready one)

(1) Soup can (It should not have ravioli, pasta, rice, or other type of grain)

(3) Sausages, pre-cooked, not frozen (these are usually found next to the bacon)

(½ lb.) Smoked fish

(1) Whole chicken rotisserie

Butter

Nuts of your choice (e.g. hazelnuts, almonds, walnuts, macadamia nuts)

Any fruit of your choice to eat one serving per day (e.g. 7 apples or 5 apples and a box of blueberries/strawberries, etc.)

Your Zero Cooking Week's Meal Plans

Sunday

For Dinner:

½ of the Rotisserie chicken
Frozen veggies

You can prepare the veggies as you like them. My suggestion is to cook them in the microwave with butter.

That evening you should boil 5 eggs and store them in the refrigerator for the rest of the week.

Monday

For Breakfast:

¼ lb. Ham
2 Boiled eggs
1 Fresh tomato

For Lunch:

Half of the Chicken rotisserie (from yesterday)
Green salad, you can add cucumber to it and any other veggie you like

For Dinner:

Italian meatballs
Frozen veggies

Tuesday

For Breakfast:

1 Apple
Nuts (1-2 handfuls)

For Lunch:

Sausage
Coleslaw

For Dinner:

Salmon
Green salad

Wednesday

For Breakfast:

2 Boiled eggs
¼ lb. Ham
Pickle

For Lunch:

Cooked chicken
Frozen veggies

For Dinner:

Beef patties
Tomato
Pickle
Green salad

Thursday

For Breakfast:

1 Apple
Nuts (1-2 handfuls)

For Lunch:

Sausage
Coleslaw

For Dinner:

Cooked chicken
Frozen veggies

Friday

For Breakfast:

Smoked fish
1 Egg
Fresh cucumber slices

For Lunch:

Shrimp in green salad

For Dinner:

Italian meatballs
Brussels sprouts

Saturday

For Breakfast:

Bacon and eggs (you could treat yourself and go to a diner for this. If you do, avoid eating bread, hash browns, home fries, pancakes, etc.)

For Lunch:

Smoked turkey

Fresh vegetable platter

For Dinner:

Soup
Sweet potato (Baked or cooked in the microwave with butter)